Praise for What Happened?

Many psychotherapists have tried to write practical and entertaining books that convey they lessons gained through their work. Saunders' work stands apart in its boldness and its iconoclasm. He is not afraid to take on the sacred cows in the field which most others tip toe around. Saunders is clearly an experienced and entertaining educator. He is less cautious and more extraverted than many others in his profession. However this is balanced by his passion in trying to be truly helpful as well as an understanding of the private worlds of his clients. There are echoes of R.D. Laing in this approach. This is especially evident in his deep respect, if not love, for his clients.

This booked is primarily written for psychotherapists and indeed any one with an active interest in how to help people with what can be broadly described as "mental health issues". It deals very much to the immediate and practical demands of dealing with individuals in crisis. It contains gems of therapeutic wisdom mined from a life time of work trying to help people in mental distress. This book represents some of the key lessons a good supervisor could convey to a new practitioner or indeed any therapist.

The author's love for his work shines through on every page. The book is in the genre of works written by psychotherapists trying to convey the challenges and the useful approaches of what they have learned through experience. The best known series of books in this area would be the series of works by Irvin Yalom.

The book is modeled on Yalom's style of conveying essential therapeutic points through the medium of case studies that are presented as dramatic stories with a significant twist – often right at the end. So in many ways it reads like a psychotherapy detective story with the author in the role of something of a Sherlock Holmes pointing out to the reader how to read a case and manage the investigation that reveals the true cause of the suffering of the patient and what is needed in terms of a remedy.

Apart from the case studies and elucidation of psychotherapeutic methods, the book provides a stinging critique of the medical model approach to mental health. This centers on a systematic debunking of the psychiatric approach and in particular the "psychiatric bible" – the Diagnostic and Statistical Manual of Mental Disorders. Here we see echoes of Thomas Szasz and his work on the "myth of mental illness".

The author goes further and deeper and suggests that the approach to mental distress needs to be based not on unknown supposed causes but on "what happened." That is, looking at the distress as being most likely the effect of various traumas and disruptions to normal psychological development. This is sometimes referred to as a "trauma informed" approach to psychotherapy.

The book also contains a comprehensive assault on the use of psychiatric medication. Medications that are commonly in use and often the only treatment provided to the many individuals appearing for a visit to the General Practitioner with a psychological problem. Saunders cites widely on a range of others who have questioned the overuse of psychiatric medications.

The book will be of interest to any one active in the field of the treatment of mental health problems. It presents a significant challenge to the orthodoxy governing the field and should lead to a productive debate aimed at enhancing the delivery of services to those in need.

– David Indemaur

WHAT HAPPENED?

What mental health is really about

Dr BILL SAUNDERS

Copyright © Bill Saunders
First published in Australia in 2021
by KMD Books
Waikiki, WA 6169

All rights reserved. No part of this book may be used or reproduced by any means, graphic, electronic, or mechanical, including photocopying, recording, taping or by any information storage retrieval system without the written permission of the copyright owner except in the case of brief quotations embodied in critical articles and reviews. Although the author and publisher have made every effort to ensure that the information in this book was correct at press time, the author and publisher do not assume and hereby disclaim any liability to any party for any loss, damage, or disruption caused by errors or omissions, whether such errors or omissions result from negligence, accident, or any other cause. This book is not intended as a substitute for the medical advice of physicians. The reader should regularly consult a physician in matters relating to his/her health and particularly with respect to any symptoms that may require diagnosis or medical attention.

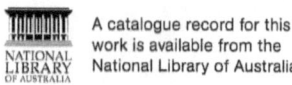 A catalogue record for this work is available from the National Library of Australia

National Library of Australia Catalogue-in-Publication data:
What Happened?/Dr Bill Saunders

ISBN: 978-0-6451353-7-4
(Paperback)

ISBN: 978-0-6451353-8-1
(eBook)

Dedication

On the day I finished writing this book, the front doorbell chimed. I opened the door. There was a gentleman standing there.

"My name is John and I have a disability and could I clean your windows? But don't hire the disability, hire the window cleaner."

So I did.

As he worked I asked him about his 'disability.'

"I'm a schizophrenic and I take a drug called resperdal. I take 7.5 milligrams every day. Do you know that drug?"

"Yes," I said, "I do. How do you find it?"

"Well, it makes me fat, but sort of stops the voices. What do you do?"

"I'm a clinical psychologist."

"It's funny, isn't it," he said, "that nobody knows what causes mental illness."

I said, "I do."

He looked at me, astonished.

I said, "What happened to you?"

He replied, "When I was six, my mum ran away from my violent father. For the next six years I was locked in my bedroom. My dad never let me out the house for six years. Is that what caused my schizophrenia?"

I said, "Yes, we know that really nasty childhoods like yours cause schizophrenia."

He said, "Thank you, I never knew that."

This book is dedicated to improving the understanding of the impact of childhood trauma upon psychological functioning and thereby (hopefully) we will improve the services we offer people with so-called 'mental illnesses.'

Foreword

On most mornings when writing this book I'd get up at first light and go for a 'clear the head run.' Running is a great way to think; especially about writing. I'd begin the run 'thinking' about how to address an issue and then somewhere in the run I would start 'having thoughts' that brought clarity.

One day, wending my way back to the beachside house that I was using as a writer's retreat, I saw the following statement written on a blackboard that normally advertised the local golf club's menu specials.

"The standard you walk past is the standard you accept."

I guiltily knew that the message applied to me. I knew that for many years, I had kept quiet about troubling things. I knew that I had, for a couple of decades at least, had a growing disquiet about how we manage mental health. But, I had remained silent. I went back that morning and I wrote with increased vigour. I toughened the book up.

The current mental health modus operandi is to consider any exhibition of emotional distress as aberrant, as a mental health disorder. Thus, we diagnose emotional pain as though it is physical pain. In classic medical model paradigm we consider what is wrong; what are the symptoms? We then apply a label, one of the currently available 250 plus mental illnesses, and medication is administered; a pill to moderate the aberrant distress.

Nowhere in this process is there any acceptance that emotions, of whatever type, from calm to catatonic or frenzied to furious, are valid emotions. The existing zeitgeist is that if you are distressed (or even worse distressing others), then the remedy is to apply a psychopharmacological response that deadens and masks your feelings. Nowhere in this paradigm is there space to acknowledge a universal psychological truth.

Which is that: all emotions are valid.

You cannot have a wrong feeling. Our feelings are never logical, and yes, you may have over reacted, or been triggered, you may even feel 'crazy,' but nonetheless such feelings are valid. You cannot have a 'wrong' feeling.

So, instead of focusing on how we assist distressed people to understand that the core of every so-called mental illness is valid emotional dysregulation (that can be managed), we tell dysregulated people that the voices they hear, the anxiety they feel, the depression they experience, are aberrant and are 'wrong.'

But what if, just for the moment, we were to see the voices, the fear and the depression as 'right.' As being the obvious, valid, real consequence of something else; with that something else being either developmental, or adulthood acquired, trauma.

It is contended in this book that in order to keep the 'your feelings are wrong' mental illness model going, psychiatry has to perpetuate four great hoaxes.

The first, is that there really are 250 plus mental illnesses that exist. In this book the contention is that they are all merely epiphenomena of trauma.

The second great hoax is that psychiatrists can reliably diagnose the 250 or so mental illnesses. Unfortunately, in psychiatry every diagnosis is nothing other than an opinion. And because opinions always vary, inter-rater reliability in the diagnosis of 'mental illness' is no better than chance.

If you see one psychiatrist, you will get one diagnosis. If you see two, the probability, at about sixty percent, is that you will get two diagnoses. But if you see three psychiatrists, you will definitely get two different diagnoses, possibly three.

Such is this variation in opinions that psychiatrists cannot reliably distinguish between schizophrenia (the purported major mental illness) and so-called personality disorders that are deemed not mental illnesses at all.

The third great hoax is that the existing two hundred and fifty plus mental illnesses have a biological base. They don't. Despite some seventy years of looking, and after billions of dollars have been spent searching for malfeasant alleles or aberrant neuro-transmitters, not a skerrick of biological evidence has been found.

So, in modern day psychiatry, the causes of all the mental illnesses, bar one, remain unknown. That one is Post Traumatic Stress Disorder (PTSD).

In modern day psychiatry there is not a single blood test, not one hard biologic endpoint, to either diagnose these biologic illnesses or sustain the claim that all mental illnesses have a biological base.

The fourth great hoax is that the 250 mental illnesses, with their purported (but yet to be discovered) biologic aetiology, can be treated effectively and efficaciously with psychopharmacology.

A psychopharmacology that was developed without any knowledge or understanding whatsoever of any underlying biological malfunction, because such malfunctions are, of course, yet to be discovered.

Thus, so-called 'anti-depressants' are not 'anti-depressants' at all, 'anti-psychotics' aren't 'anti-psychotics' and the so-called 'mood stabilizers' are either 'anti-epilepsy' drugs or 'anti-psychotics,' that aren't of course 'anti-psychotics,' because we still don't know the biologic aetiology of psychosis; though we do know that psychosis is a consequence of trauma.

The compelling evidence is that all psychopharmacology changes your brain chemistry, even though there's absolutely no evidence that your brain chemistry is in any way aberrant. Thus, you will get nasty side effects, develop tolerance, and if you cease using 'psych meds,' you will have nasty withdrawals (oops, sorry, 'discontinuation syndrome.')

And the accumulating evidence is that they don't work; but more about that in the book.

As I ran past the sign that morning, I knew that I had walked past a too low standard of care for people with mental health disorders (emotional dysregulation) for too long. Hence this book.

It was time to stand up and promulgate a different discourse, which, in a nutshell, is "What Happened To You?" rather than the false psychiatric rhetoric of "What Is Wrong With You?"

And the acceptance of a style of care, trauma-informed psychotherapy, that directly addresses the absolute aetiology of mental health; one's capacity to regulate one's emotions.

Bill Saunders
Trigg March 2021

Contents

Chapter One
What's wrong with "What's Wrong With You?" 1

Chapter Two
What happened to you? 21

Chapter Three
Dramatic fine spies's 34

Chapter Four
The teacher 53

Chapter Five
Once were reptiles 62

Chapter Six
Getting out of jail 74

Chapter Seven
The woman who drowned 91

Chapter Eight
Perfect psychosis 103

Chapter Nine
"I want to die." 116

Chapter Ten
The man who wanted to kill and eat me 126

Chapter Eleven
Pixie packs them in 135

Chapter Twelve
You can't go past a vagina 142

Chapter Thirteen
Addiction doesn't exist 152

Chapter Fourteen
Must get it right 162

Chapter Fifteen
"I'd slap the little cunt" 167

Chapter Sixteen
The apple of his mother's eye 171

Chapter Seventeen
Running on empty 177

Chapter Eighteen
Some reflections on being a psychotherapist 182

Chapter Nineteen
Conclusion 186

Chapter Twenty
Finale 189

Acknowledgements 194

Glossary 196

References 200

Chapter One

What's wrong with "What's Wrong With You?"

How you understand something dictates how you respond to it. In the world of mental health, there are various paradigms of understanding; the dominant one being the "What's Wrong With You?" model. In this essentially psychiatric perspective, the key to responding to mental health problems is to assess, diagnose then treat the sufferer for their "purportedly" biological mental illness. This treatment is unfailingly psychopharmacological; a pill for every mental ill.

But, there is an emerging, increasingly persuasive and well-substantiated paradigm, that this book contends is now sufficiently robust to challenge the dominant discourse. It is the, "What Happened To You?" model.

Here, the understanding is that "What Happened To You," especially as a child, is critical in the determination of your mental health. In this model, the intervention is trauma-informed psychotherapy. From this perspective the "What's Wrong With You?" model is seen as fatally flawed and detrimental to the wellbeing of people with mental health issues; numbing or masking emotional pain with medication is simply not acceptable.

Significantly, in the "What Happened To You?" model, *there is no diagnosis*. Importantly, unlike the "What's Wrong With You?" model, the aetiology of mental ill health *is* known; the myriad of so-called "mental illnesses" are manifestations of childhood neglect and/or abuse.

This statement is driven by the experience of being a Clinical Psychologist who was trained in, and fully believed in, the "What's Wrong With You?" model for decades. However, gradually, through an amalgam of clinical experience, research, reading, exposure to different interventions and a very real dissatisfaction with the limitations of biological psychiatry, I have transferred my allegiance to the "What Happened To You?" model.

To start with, I want to quickly (and hopefully effectively) demolish the "What's Wrong With You" model.

In doing so, I understand that I am challenging the pre-eminent model on which governments spend billions of dollars each year, especially in the Western world. It is also very effectively championed by the psychopharmacological industry ("Big Pharma") and, of course, the profession of psychiatry.

I also understand that one chapter is not going to change the world. However, hopefully, the following will cause you to pause and perhaps reconsider the possibilities.

There is a passage in Lewis Carroll's *Alice in Wonderland* that I delighted in, when I read it as a nine or ten year old. It goes like this:

> *Alice laughed. "There's no use trying," she said: "One cannot believe impossible things."*
> *"I dare say you haven't had much practice," said the Queen. "When I was your age, I always did it for half an hour a day. Why sometimes I've believed as many as six impossible things before breakfast."*

So, let's begin the demolition of the "What's Wrong With You?" model, with an invitation for you to believe six impossible things before the end of the chapter. Here we go.

The maxim of the Clinical Psychology master's course that I completed many years ago was "get the diagnosis right and the right treatment will follow."

There was a built-in corollary which was, "if the patient failed to improve it was because the diagnosis was wrong." Such was the emphasis on diagnosis.

Some twenty-odd years later when I ended up in charge of a Clinical Psychology course, we were mandated by our accreditors to include specific teaching on the recognition of mental health disorders and their specific management. Diagnosis was again seen as the key to appropriate intervention.

In clinical medicine, diagnosis works like this. You present at your doctor's, describe your symptoms, and the GP will send you off for X-rays, or scans, or blood tests, to confirm his or her hunch about what ails you. In clinical medicine there are, in this diagnostic process, hard end points and *biologic markers* for diagnosis.

Let's take an exemplar. The patient, let's make him a fifty-seven-year-old male, turns up at his doctor's talking about an urgency to urinate regularly, especially at night, but has difficulty in doing so. The doctor will have his or her suspicions as to what is wrong. Could it be prostate cancer?

WHAT HAPPENED?

A rectal examination of the patient's prostate gland may occur, but a Prostate Specific Antigen (PSA) blood test will also be undertaken. Let's say the rectal examination is equivocal, as is, when it comes back, the PSA score. The patient has a PSA score of 6.2. This is an elevated score, but is not of itself conclusive that the patient has prostate cancer. So, the doctor may decide to run another PSA test in six to eight weeks, but in the meantime prescribes an antibiotic just in case the prostate is infected.

The second PSA blood test comes back at 9.2. Not good news at all, but still not certain news. However, on the basis of the results so far an MRI of the prostate is warranted. This shows several cellular abnormalities, so a biopsy of the prostate is undertaken. Under pathological examination the results come back revealing that tissue from the prostate is abnormal and in the two worst areas the abnormalities are scored as being 9/10; very significant abnormality. The patient has prostate cancer. Treatment then follows.

All the way through this process, the doctor's initial opinion was evaluated against independent objective testing. Diagnosis was achieved through the use of a specific physiological test, scans and a biological procedure. The original doctor's hunch that the patient had prostate cancer was independently confirmed.

Unfortunately, in psychiatry, and in the management of mental health disorders, there are no hard endpoints at all. There are no independent biological markers whatsoever. There is no independent third-party confirmation. Despite all the breakthrough claims made for biological psychiatry, not one definitive test exists.

In psychiatry this difficulty is, in fact, well-recognised. For example, in 2013, at the time of the publication of the 5th Diagnostic and Statistical Manual of Mental Disorders (known colloquially as the DSM 5 - the psychiatric diagnosis bible), the President of the American Psychiatric Association (APA), psychiatrist Jeffrey Lieberman, noted that genetics and biomarkers were not included in DSM 5.0 as there was not yet sufficient evidence for their inclusion.

Interestingly, on the publication of DSM 5.0, Dr. Tom Insel, the head of the National Institute for Mental Health (NIMH), the lead American mental health research agency, commented that patients deserved better than the DSM 5.0.

Insel then advocated for a new diagnostic system based on bio markers, neurobiology, genetics and brain functioning. He wanted a precision medicine approach to mental illness. That, in keeping with the zeitgeist of the need for independent diagnostics, was both warranted and laudable.

However, four years later, Insel wrote that while he had spent thirteen years in his position at NIMH looking into the genetics and neuroscience behind mental disorders, and despite research undertaken during that time to the tune of around $20 billion, he acknowledged that they hadn't reduced the rates of suicide or hospitilisations.

A startling admission, a very concerning admission, and one that confirms that there are still no biological markers for any of the mental health disorders, because the *biological* causes of mental illness remain unknown. This is important. In the dominant model of mental illness, the cause, of all but one, remain unknown. Interestingly, the one that is known is Post Traumatic Stress Disorder (PTSD), which isn't of course biological, but rather a consequence of an adverse experience, or "What Happened To You?"

The failure to know what causes the 250 plus other mental illnesses may be because the biological causes have not been found yet. Or, could it be that they are not biologically caused? Unfortunately, you can never prove a negative, so the expensive (fruitless?) search goes on.

Today the diagnosis of a mental health disorder is, just like a hundred years ago, nothing other than an opinion. "I think you've got bipolar," "I think you have schizophrenia," "I think you have an anxiety disorder," "I think you have depression."

It may be an informed opinion based on training and experience, but an opinion nonetheless. The trouble is that people's opinions differ, often markedly.

To demonstrate the precariousness of this complete lack of hard endpoints, of biological markers, of anything resembling objective science on the management of mental health, and also remembering the Queen's conversation with Alice, here is the first impossible thing to believe about the "What's Wrong With You?" model, that I'd like you to believe.

Impossible thing to believe #1

Consider the case of Mr. Anders Breivik. Mr. Breivik was the man who, in 2011, exploded a bomb in Oslo then drove to an island off the coast of Norway and shot sixty-nine young people dead. Mr. Breivik was arrested by the police. His justification for his slayings was that Norway was becoming contaminated by immigrants.

As part of the preparation for Breivik's trial, the prosecution had Mr. Breivik interviewed by two independent psychiatrists. After an extensive assessment, they concluded that Mr. Breivik was suffering from schizophrenia. He was therefore not responsible for his actions because it was deemed that on the day of the shooting he was actively psychotic (mad).

If you refer to page ninety-nine of the current psychiatric diagnostic bible (DSM 5.0) you will find that there are five key symptoms of schizophrenia.

These are:

WHAT HAPPENED?

- Delusions
- Hallucinations
- Disorganised speech
- Grossly disorganised or catatonic behaviour
- Negative symptoms such as avolition or diminished emotional expression

However, as this diagnosis became known it became increasingly unpopular. Even Mr. Breivik didn't like it. So the defence got two different psychiatrists to assess Mr. Breivik. After an extensive assessment, they concluded that the original diagnosis was incorrect.

In their opinion, Mr. Breivik had an anti-social personality disorder. On page 659 of DSM 5.0 you will find the diagnostic criteria for anti-social personality disorder. There are seven key features and you need three or more to earn the diagnosis. They are as follows:

- A failure to conform to social norms with respect to lawful behaviour
- Deceitfulness
- Impulsivity and a failure to plan ahead
- Reckless disregard for self or others
- Irritability and aggressiveness
- Consistent irresponsibilty
- Lack of remorse

If you compare the criteria for schizophrenia and those for anti-social personality disorder, it is clear that none of the diagnostic criteria overlap. The two disorders are literally as different as chalk and cheese. Yet, both teams of psychiatrists were convinced as to the correctness of their totally different diagnoses.

But, then again, people are usually disposed to think that their opinions are right.

This was an important finding because it meant that Mr. Breivik could be tried for his crimes. He was bad, not mad. This second opinion stood, and Mr. Breivik was sentenced to the Norwegian equivalent of life in prison.

So how can this be? How can schizophrenia, which is considered to be *the* major mental health "illness," be confused with a disorder of personality? Especially, as personality disorders are, in the DSMs, not conceptualised as being mental health "illnesses" at all.

Surely the basic, fundamental test of any diagnostic system is to be able to determine which people have an "illness" and which do not?

The Breivik case demonstrates that the current psychiatric diagnosis system failed this basic test.

Yet, the Breivik case was not really surprising. His situation was mirrored totally in a 1970s study where psychiatrists in Canada, the USA and Britain were asked to independently diagnose case studies.

In one case, Case F, fifty-three percent of the 250 American psychiatrists in the study concluded that the patient had schizophrenia; a one in two agreement rate, which you might consider surprisingly low. After all, schizophrenia is deemed to be the major mental health illness.

However, it got worse. Of the 115 Canadian psychiatrists involved in the study, only twenty-seven percent agreed that Case F was schizophrenic; a one in three agreement rate. If you put the American and the Canadian psychiatrists together then the agreement rate for the 365 psychiatrists involved was forty-five percent. Thus, the interrater agreement rate in the diagnosis of whether Case F was schizophrenic was now below one in two.

If you toss a coin 365 times the number of "heads" that come up will be, purely by chance, somewhere between forty-five and fifty-five percent of the coin tosses.

And still, the results got even worse.

Of the 194 British psychiatrists only two percent, yes, two percent, that's four British psychiatrists, considered Case F to have schizophrenia; a one in fifty agreement rate. The majority of British psychiatrists considered that, in their opinion, Case F had a personality disorder.

Thus, for the entire study, the inter-rater agreement on whether Case F had schizophrenia was thirty percent. The agreement rate on whether Case F had a personality disorder was thirty-seven percent and "other" diagnoses were thirty-three percent.

How can this possibly be? How can the most major of mental health illnesses, schizophrenia, only be recognised by a third of over 550 practising psychiatrists?

If you take a pack of cards and remove, say, all the diamonds, so that you have three categories (hearts, clubs and spades or metaphorically schizophrenia, personality disorder and other) and you then shuffle the cards, put them face down into three piles, the number of spades, clubs and hearts you will have in each pile will be somewhere in the thirty percents, purely by chance.

So, impossible thing to believe number one: based on the 1970s study, and the fact that nothing in the way in which diagnosis is achieved has subsequently changed, psychiatrists cannot reliably distinguish people with the mental illness of schizophrenia from those with non-mental illnesses such as personality disorders. Indeed, they do no better than chance.

Impossible thing to believe #2

Diagnostic reliability is essentially when two people see the same thing, say, a giraffe, and they independently and without prompting agree that it is a giraffe. Then if you extend the test out to include, say, elephants, cheetahs, leopards, tigers, lions and chipmunks, and again ask two or more independent witnesses what they see, it is possible to determine what the inter-rater reliability rate is. Obviously one hundred per cent is optimum, but it is seldom, if ever, achieved. When asked, human beings cannot unanimously agree which day of the week it is; apparently ninety per cent for day of the week is very good.

So when it comes to psychiatric diagnosis, just how good are psychiatrists at agreeing about what they see?

Well it depends who you ask. Jeffrey Lieberman, former President of the APA and author of the acclaimed book *Shrinks* has written: "Mental disorders are abnormal, enduring, harmful, treatable, feature a biological component and can be *reliably* diagnosed."

Unfortunately, in my opinion, his assertion of reliability is, unreliable. Similarly, the assertion of a biological component is contradicted, as there is a pronouncement in the same book that no biological causes have been found (yet) for any of the 260 plus mental illnesses outlined in DSM 5.0.

Here is why, I believe, his claim is unreliable.

With the advent of DSM III in 1980 and its putatively new and improved diagnostic categories, considerable effort was made to address the diagnostic reliability problems identified above; that very troublesome Canadian, USA and UK study was undertaken in the early 1970s and based on DSM II.

DSM III was deemed to be a considerable improvement on its 1960's predecessor DSM II. As a way of addressing the known difficulties of opinion-based diagnostics, the principal redress was to define clear criteria for each mental illness. The man behind this work was Dr. Robert Spitzer, who was given the monumental task of "creating" the diagnostic criteria for all of the eventual 256 mental health "illnesses" that came to be in DSM III. It took him six years to do so.

A structured clinical interview (known as the SCID) was also created based on the same diagnostic criteria outlined in DSM III and then its revision in 1986, the DSM III R. After the introduction of the SCID, the DSM IIIR was put to the test.

This study involved some six hundred patients, attending five sites in America and one in Germany, being interviewed by twenty-five clinicians, all of whom had been trained in the use of the SCID. Each patient was separately interviewed by two clinicians and an inter-rater agreement score was then determined.

However, in cases of diagnostic disagreement, the two interviewers were allowed to reconsider their original opinions and were *invited* "to arrive at consensual diagnoses."

Interestingly, the authors did acknowledge that the little device of allowing dissenting raters to arrive at consensus by post-interview consultation may have artificially raised reliability. Now that's a very *real* probability, but they then dismissed this probability because they considered that the achieved inter-rater reliability values were too *low* for this too have occurred.

How does that work? I have a little suspicion that if the researchers had not "consulted" in this way then the achieved values may have been even lower.

From a research perspective, this is a highly dubious practice, but nonetheless the best overall reliability scores the raters could achieve for their "independent" diagnoses was a kappa score of 0.61. (A kappa score is a statistical measure of reliability).

For this study, Dr. Spitzer determined that a kappa score of 0.7 and above was "high," from 0.5 to 0.7 "fair" and below 0.5 "poor."

This categorisation is in itself of interest because in earlier work, Dr. Spitzer had declared that a kappa score of 0.7 was "only satisfactory," and below 0.7 "poor."

This lowering the bar, meant what was claimed as "fair" reliability in this study, would, in previous research, have been labelled as "poor."

That is of itself interesting. Additionally, and also problematically, the lead researcher on this independent study, Janet Williams, later became Dr. Spitzer's wife. Would it be outrageous to suggest that the impartiality of the research team was in doubt?

Just to confound the results a little further, another sleight of hand occurred. The definition of what a match was, well, let's call it generous. In DSM III, there are 265 possible reliable diagnoses, but in this research these 265 possibilities were collapsed into classes.

It's like testing people to name specific types of cars, such as a Volkswagen Golf GTi, a Range Rover Sport, or a Mazda 3, but all you need to claim that they both called it the same thing, is for them to say "oh, it's a Mazda," "it's a Land Rover," or "it's a Volkswagen." Now that's easier. Thus, agreement as to the same *class* of diagnosis was deemed a match even if the two raters disagreed, for example, on the type of personality disorder that a patient had. Thus, as long as they both said, "it's a Mazda," despite one saying "it's a Mazda 3," and the other "it's a Mazda CX 30," – then it's a match!

From my perspective, I wonder if that could also have artificially inflated the achieved reliability values.

A two dollar coin and a five cent coin are both money, yet we certainly expect our banks and our accountants to do better than considering them both the same.

If this was not damning enough, there was another awkward finding. The sample of patients was drawn from six sites. Four of these were clinical units, but two were not. These non-psychiatric sites were a community medical facility and a sample of anxious, worried or depressed people recruited by advertising in community newspapers. The inter-rater reliability Kappa scores achieved here were 0.32 and 0.38 respectively.

I think that however you jiggle it, these results would fall in the "very poor" or "totally unsatisfactory" categories.

The thing is, as people become more distressed, they become more conspicuous. Diagnosing the acute, severe cases seems easier, but only to a certain point.

Finally, and most tellingly, all the raters in this study were trained using a Standardised Clinical Interview (the SCID). This is a flawed model. No every day, ordinarily practising psychiatrist ever uses such a thing. The very device invented to improve reliability in clinical practice is totally eschewed by the profession it was invented for.

To be fair to the authors of the above study, they did finally admit defeat: "Prior to this study we expected higher reliability values. We are at a loss to explain why this was not the case."

For me, there is one very simple explanation, which is that the 265 disorders identified in the DSM III are not mutually exclusive, that is, they are not separate disorders at all. They blur into each other because they are merely variations on a theme. They are different manifestations of the same aetiology: childhood neglect and/or abuse.

Interestingly, in the lead up to the production of the next DSM (DSM IV) the APA received funding from an independent charitable foundation to undertake a new reliability study. Tellingly, although the data collection phase of the project was completed, the findings of the study were never published. The project's director said at the time that the APA ran out of money.

That is surprising, because as a former researcher, I am all too aware that in any research project a budget has to be submitted at the time of application for any grant. It is always the data collection, not the analysis, that is the most expensive part, and if things go astray, then the budget can be blown. Running out of money in the analysis stage is less common, and even if you do, funding bodies are often sympathetic to valid over-runs. If this very important project had run out of money, then surely in the interests of science additional funding could have been sought from either the original funders or elsewhere.

Indeed, given that the sales of DSM III and IIIR generated in excess of $25 million for the APA (in 1980s value), then surely any shortfall could have been met by the APA themselves. Especially as, if the results had been as good as has been subsequently claimed, that would have further strengthened the marketing of later editions of the DSMs. It is reported that over one million copies of DSM IV were sold for an impressive $80 million. (DSM IV was published, the study about its reliability wasn't). Surely there would have been something in the kitty to fund an analysis of the earlier obtained results?

Then there is just the small matter of the field trials that occurred in the lead up to DSM 5.0.

As for all previous DSM editions, the methods used to assess reliability were claimed to reflect "current standards for psychiatric investigation. Independent interviews by two different clinicians trained in the diagnoses, each prompted by a computerised checklist."

Well such methods may reflect current *research* practice, but as will be apparent, they do not reflect everyday *clinical* practice where a single practitioner makes the diagnosis without any help from any computer check-list or special pre-study diagnostic training. The only training in diagnosis in real life practice is what psychiatrists were exposed to when studying for admission to psychiatry. That could, of course, have been anywhere from five to fifty years ago. So although the study may look good from a research perspective such work clearly lacks ethnographic validity; that is it fails to replicate real life.

So how did the field trials for the next DSM go? Well according to the researchers they went very well. They even claimed that at last in psychiatric practice "a rose is a rose is a rose."

Ah, unless you have a generalised anxiety disorder, the inter-rater kappa score was 0.2 (remember Dr. Bob Spitzer claiming that anything below 0.7 was "poor"), so for anxiety, a rose is a dandelion or perhaps a cactus.

For the illness of major depression the raters could only achieve 0.28 (a rose is a cabbage or a banana perhaps), and anti-social personality disorder came in at 0.26, (a rose is a geranium or a fir tree).

Interestingly, the authors also claimed that their research showed "the problem in distinguishing schizophrenia, bipolar disorder, and schizoaffective disorder—a prior, vexed issue—has largely been resolved, and all three conditions have good Kappa statistics."

Excellent, except the purported good kappa statistics, were 0.46, 0.56 and 0.50 respectively. The researchers achieved so-called good kappas not by improvements in their diagnostic categories but by the redefining of "good Kappa" down from "above 0.7" to 0.45.

Furthermore, these "good" results were only obtained by the artifice of having specially trained for the study psychiatric researchers aided by a computer checklist.

Given the above, the following comment by trenchant critic of psychiatry, Bonnie Burstow, seems considered and very reasonable. She noted that the claims of "high reliability, indeed of improved reliability, in short is not a reality, but a discursive product."

Two psychologists, Kutchins and Kirk, after reviewing the literature relating to diagnostic reliability concluded, "the DSM revolution in reliability has been a revolution of rhetoric not reality."

I could be blunter, in fact, I will be. The claims of improved reliability, even reliability per se, are unreliable.

So what does Dr. Bob Spitzer, the man who set himself the task of improving the reliability of psychiatric diagnosis, really think? Well, this is what he wrote:

"To say that we've solved the reliability problem is just not true. It's been improved. But if you're in a situation with a general clinician, it's certainly not very good. There's still a real problem, and it's not clear how to solve the problem."

So impossible thing to believe number two: psychiatrists never have, and still cannot, *reliably* diagnose any of the purported "mental illnesses."

Impossible thing to believe #3

If the above was not confronting enough then there is the American study in which a Professor of Psychology at Stanford University, one Dr. Rosenhan, sent eight stooge patients (one being himself), who were not psychotic, to psychiatric hospitals in the USA where they pretended to be psychotic. (They went to 12 hospitals!)

They behaved normally, but said they had a voice in their head that said things like "thud" or "empty." All were admitted. To be fair they looked dishevelled, having not showered or shaved for a few days. Seven were diagnosed as being schizophrenic and were "treated" with anti-psychotics. After admission they all said their voices were no longer present.

However, they then encountered a problem. They couldn't get out. Not only did the psychiatrists misdiagnose them in the first place, they then couldn't diagnose that they were sane.

Eventually, as all patients do, they got out; though one was incarcerated for seven weeks.

Rosenhan wrote about his experiences in a paper delightfully titled "On Being Sane in Insane Places."

Needless to say there were great protests from the psychiatric profession. One outraged hospital director even challenged Rosenhan to send them more fakes. He agreed. Later, the hospital proudly reported they had detected 41 fakes.

Yet none had been sent.

It is acknowledged that this study has recently been severely criticised and it has even been claimed that the study never really occurred as Rosenhan described (for example see Scull 2019), but that does not detract from the very premise of the study, that diagnosis even of the major mental illnesses, is a matter of individual judgement, and that because nothing has changed this study could be replicated today.

Thus, impossible thing to believe number three: psychiatrists cannot today reliably distinguish mad people from sane people; or sane ones from mad ones.

Impossible thing to believe #4

This opinion-based diagnostic process has, not surprisingly given its critics, come under enormous and expensive review and re-appraisal.

From the 1950s onwards attempts have been made to improve, refine and make better the psychiatric bible. So DSM 1 spawned DSMs 2, 3, 4, and recently 5. Sorry, that's not right. Officially the DSMs are I, II, III, IV and then 5. Using Latin numerals for the first four obviously gave gravitas. Yet, for the fifth revision it became DSM 5.0 because, according to the then Chairman of the APA, making it 5.0 would then allow 5.1, 5.2, 5.3, just like software upgrades, so the right tone of modern, continual, scientific improvement was set.

Such is the marketing inherent in the process of psychiatric diagnostics.

Over time, to help psychiatrists get it right, some disorders (such as homosexuality, alcohol dependence syndrome, and paranoid schizophrenia) have been removed, most others, clarified and refined.

Actually, the removal of homosexuality as a mental health disorder is of considerable interest because it is a marker of how in psychiatry the "what is and what is not a mental illness" process works.

In DSM I homosexuality was a personality disorder, in DSM II a sexual deviance, but in DSM III homosexuality was removed. Well, sort of removed. To pander to those psychiatrists who wanted homosexuality to remain, it was replaced by "sexual orientation disturbance." These changes were made by members of the APA's Research Council taking a vote. Yes, a vote.

During that event, the reliable, valid, previous mental illness of homosexuality from DSM I and DSM II was voted out; 5854 to 3810.

Thus, it seems, whether something is a mental illness or is not a mental illness, is actually a political enterprise.

Though, as outlined below, on some occasions the creation/invention of a mental illness is an individual exercise.

In 2005, author Alix Spiegel wrote an article published in the *New Yorker* magazine, about Roger Peel and Paul Luisada. In 1974, they were both psychiatrists at St. Elizabeth's Hospital in Washington D.C. In a paper published that year, they used the phrase "hysterical pyschoses" to describe two kinds of patients; those who were compelled to visit an emergency department without genuine physical or psychological problems, and those who had short periods of delusion and hallucination after an extreme traumatic event. It seems that Spitzer, on reading the paper, requested to meet with Peel and Luisada in Washington. Alix Spiegel goes on to explain that after forty minutes of conversation, the three decided that "hysterical psychoses" was actually two different disorders and labelled them "brief reactive psychosis," and "factitious disorder." As told to Spiegel, Spitzer then asked for a typewriter and drafted the definitions right then, during that meeting.

Both factitious disorder and brief reactive psychosis were included in the DSM III with only minor adjustments.

Thus, mental illnesses are not, as in real medicine, discovered, they are invented, sometimes by one man talking to two colleagues. Both these "mental illnesses" are still in DSM 5.0.

Mental illnesses are popularised and socially constructed. Voted in, voted out, changed and adapted and then voted on again. So, a bit like the cat in Alice in Wonderland, mental illnesses "appear out of nowhere, bewilder us for a while and then mysteriously disappear."

In essence, we have a group of specialists with different opinions being asked their opinion on which opinions are right.

The extent of this "social construction" of mental illness, can be seen by merely reflecting on the number of mental illnesses there actually are.

In 1952, and the DSM I, there were 106 bona fide mental illnesses, but by 1968 and the DSM II this number had risen to 182. In 1980 and the DSM III there were 265 reliable, valid and definite diagnoses, but just fourteen years later in the DSM IV there were 297.

So, it is official, the world is going mad.

Then, lo and behold, in DSM 5.0, despite the inclusion of fourteen new disorders, such devilish nasties as "disinhibited social engagement disorder," "excoriation disorder," "hypersexual disorder," "hoarding disorder" and "social connection withdrawal disorder," the overall number *reduced* back down to DSM III levels at 265 definite reliable, categorical, politically created and voted on illnesses.

What is interesting about the new mental illnesses outlined above is that all of them are from my clinical experience the result, or impact, of childhood trauma.

The reduction in the number of mental illnesses in DSM 5.0 was a direct result of public and media criticism over the escalation in numbers in DSM IV and was achieved by collapsing some previously totally reliable and valid disorders, such past guaranteed stalwarts as "paranoid schizophrenia" down into the overarching category of schizophrenia and a myriad of literally odd disorders being collapsed into "autism."

What is fascinating is that the chairman of the DSM 5.0 task force actually promised, prior to the publication of DSM 5.0, that there would be no increase in the number of mental illnesses; politics determining psychiatric practice yet again.

Nevertheless, in the past seventy years (DSM I was published in 1952), there has been a 150 percent increase in the number of mental illnesses.

For those wishing to explore this topic more, James Davies' book *Cracked,* Nikolas Rose's *Our Psychiatric Future*, Bonnie Burstow's *Psychiatry and the Business of Madness,* and Richard Bentall's *Doctoring the Mind* are all compelling indictments of the process of inventing mental illnesses and having an opinion-based process as to "What's Wrong With You?"

So what's the lesson of all of this? Well, if you are a practising psychiatrist, you probably have to play the game of believing that there are mental illnesses, so you can think "What's Wrong With You?" and treat such illnesses. However dubious that enterprise may be.

However, if you are a non-medical therapist, may I suggest you don't play "The What's Wrong With You" game at all? Being a therapist, psychotherapist, counsellor, social worker, psychologist, chaplain, a case manager, child protection worker, group home worker, or drug counsellor, is not medicine, is not psychiatry. So why follow a psychiatric/biological model? Let's just leave them to it. After all, there are more of us than there are of them. If we eschew the "What's Wrong With You?" paradigm, if we talk to each other about our clients as human beings who have unfortunately as children experienced not enough of the right stuff, and often too much of the wrong stuff, then we can leave the "What's Wrong With You?" model to psychiatry.

I have made it a practice to never engage with a psychiatrist in any diagnostic debate. I just agree with them. They will, in all probability, later change their minds. If the patient sees a different psychiatrist then the near certainty is that they will get another opinion, sorry, diagnosis, anyway.

So, impossible thing to believe number four: the 265 currently real mental illnesses are not real at all. They are social constructions that may or may not be with us in the future. What they all are, in fact, are different manifestations of the impact of childhood neglect and abuse.

Impossible thing to believe #5

There is another fundamental problem with the "What's Wrong with You?" model. Diagnosis is supposed to be the driver of treatment. In real medicine if you have septicaemia you get prescribed an antibiotic. If you have breast cancer an antibiotic is of no use, surgery and perhaps chemotherapy is the call. If you have hypertension, an anti-hypertensive is, as I know, the way to go.

The majority of physical (biologically discovered) illnesses have a specific treatment that addresses the known causation. There are literally thousands of illnesses (circa 10,000) and thousands of specific treatments (possibly 6000). The shortfall is due to some biologically diagnosable conditions having, as yet, no known treatments. A ratio of, at worst, two to one.

However, psychiatrists currently have 265 illnesses, but only have seven, or perhaps eight, specific treatments. Really, at the absolute best, just eight: a ratio of thirty-three to one.

The treatments that are available to psychiatrists are as follows:

(i) the prescription of an "anti-depressant" (that isn't really an anti-depressant at all – more later on that).
(ii) the prescription of an "anti-psychotic" (that isn't really an anti-psychotic at all – more later).
(iii) or the prescription os a "mood stabilizer" (yes, you get it, they aren't really mood stabilizers at all).
(iv) they actually can prescribe an anti-anxiety drug. There are real anti-anxiety drugs (benzodiazepines drugs such as Valium, Xanax or Serapax). The only trouble is that they all rapidly cause psychological and physical dependence and since the late 1990s the prescription of these has been severely called into question.

So, after the so-called "anti-depressants," "anti-psychotics," "mood stabilizers" and anxiolytics, there are, at best, four more treatment options in the psychiatrist's locker:

(v) the prescription of drugs for drug dependence. These psychopharmacologies include such things as Methadone, Antabuse, Baclofen and Subutex.
(vi) drugs to manage things such as the "behavioural disorders," medications such as dexamphetamine, Ritalin or Strattera.
(vii) a catch-all group of different drugs for diverse disorders such as Cyproterone to reduce the sexual capacity of sex offenders, (of very doubtful utility), and Donepezil to manage/palliate the dementias.
(viii) the use of physical treatments such as Electroconvulsive Therapy (ECT) and, more recently, Transcranial Magnetic Stimulation (TMS). The therapeutic benefit of ECT is zero and although TMS has been highly touted, the jury is still out on whether it actually, really, works.

As an aside, the history of ECT is of interest. In the USA, the use of ECT as a legitimate therapy for the treatment of depression has never been subject to any trials. Its introduction as an approved therapy was achieved by Dr. Max Fink, a psychiatrist who sat on an APA task force on ECT that reported to the Federal Drug Administration (FDA). Because ECT is not a drug there was no requirement for any double blind clinical trial to be undertaken.

The fact that the psychiatrist who promoted ECT as being safe and effective had a licence to manufacture and sell ECT machines did not seem to be problematic.

The reality of ECT has been succinctly addressed by Dr. Bonnie Burstow who, after reviewing all the research evidence, concluded that, ECT is a dangerous treatment that can damage the brain, impair memory and induce global cognitive dysfunction. And, in fact, has no positive outcome.

The most damning evidence is that ECT is as effective in managing depression when the patient believes they have had ECT (when they have not) as when they really have had ECT.

However, the real point here is what's the point of having in excess of over 260 mental illnesses if there are only eight specific treatments?

And here's another problem. Because of the above noted dependency inducing and horrible withdrawal profile of benzodiazepines (anti-anxiety drugs), the most common response by GPs and psychiatrists alike, in the management of so called "anxiety disorders," is to prescribe either an "anti-depressant," usually Pristiq or Lexapro, or even more peculiar, an "anti-psychotic." Seroquel is the current favourite. And, notwithstanding a raft of side effects, patients report that their anxiety is reduced.

How can this be? If "anti-depressants" were really "anti-depressants," and if "anxiety disorders" were really a distinct "mental illness" separate from the "mental illness" of "depression," then a drug made for the illness of "depression" surely couldn't/wouldn't work for someone with the distinct and separate illness of "anxiety." It would be like me taking an antibiotic for my hypertension.

This is a very interesting inference, considering that "anti-depressants" are now the most commonly prescribed drug in the management of anxiety disorders. Is it that rather than "anxiety" and "depression" being very separate, distinct illnesses, maybe they are not? Is it just possible that they are merely different manifestations of the same thing?

There's that idea again. Childhood neglect and/or abuse have a raft of varying detrimental impacts on psychological functioning. The notion that there are clear cases of depression and distinct cases of anxiety is, in the clinical world, just not true. People who have been neglected and physically or sexually abused attend therapy reporting a myriad of overlapping features or symptoms. It is only this overlap that can possibly explain why the prescribing of a so-called "anti-depressant" to a so-called "anxious person" is at all useful.

There is, of course, a further group of treatments that most psychiatrists use very sparingly. That, of course, is psychotherapy. Most psychiatrists prefer to leave that to others. Yet psychotherapy works better and is more effective than psychiatric medications.

This is a bold assertion, I know, but it is assertion based on lots of evidence.

For example, in a meta-analysis (an add-lots-of-studies-together study) of psychiatric outcome undertaken by Schedler in 2010, psychotherapy was found to be at least three times more effective than psychopharmacology. When specific types of more complex therapy were included, this jumped out to an effect size of six-fold greater effectiveness.

The eminent American psychiatrist and psychotherapist Irvin Yalom has written that he is very adept at diagnosis. He prides himself that at the end of the first session he can, with confidence, nail a label to the patient's mast. However, he continued to note, by the sixth session he had completely forgotten what his diagnosis was, because by then he was working with a human being and diagnosis was irrelevant. Yalom has perspicaciously written, "Labels do violence to people. You can't treat the label; you have to treat the person behind the label."

Impossible thing to believe number five: in mental health, diagnosis doesn't matter.

Impossible thing to believe #6

Now for a salutary tale, one that is totally true, and that very early on in my career as a clinical psychologist, taught me a lesson that I ignored for years. This is the case of James McFadden, affectionately known to all as "Wee Jimmy."

In 1976, every Thursday evening, a team of us from the hospital I worked in, a Community Nurse, an Occupational Therapist, a Psychiatric Registrar (trainee psychiatrist) and me, ventured into Clydebank (a very deprived town to the west of Glasgow), and worked in a local community hall at a drop-in mental health service. We all volunteered our time. The service was free.

Looking back it was revolutionary, but at the time it was just something we decided (after a Friday night in a pub) to do. The Council of Alcoholism (a local NGO) came on board and we also started to run groups for people with alcohol dependence. Word spread.

One Thursday a man turned up and said that he was very worried about his brother Jimmy. Jimmy wouldn't leave the house.

Later that same night, a psychiatric registrar and I went to see Jimmy (now there's community mental health in action).

We sat and talked to Jimmy. He hadn't been out of his house for six weeks. He was scared to be outside alone. He didn't like crowds, he got his brother to do his shopping and he didn't like to go on trains and buses. He hadn't driven his car for a year. He was visibly anxious and shaking.

The psychiatrist and I agreed. Jimmy was agoraphobic. He was given a one-off script for some Valium to help with his anxiety. We asked Jimmy to get his brother to bring him to our community clinic the following week. He did so. I saw him and we agreed that every Thursday he would come to the community clinic, but as part of his treatment I also expected him to come to the hospital clinic in which I worked.

We agreed a plan of action. We would do one session of talk and one of walk. At that time the benchmark treatment for agoraphobia was graduated exposure therapy. I explained to Jimmy that the key feature of agoraphobia was the fear of being outside alone. Thus, the cognitive behavioural treatment we would use was for me to take him out for a walk and gradually invite him, with my support, to walk further and further on his own. I noted that this would, over time, extend to him using public transport.

Our Thursday night psychotherapy sessions were immensely agreeable. Jimmy was a freelance journalist and was a fascinating local historian. His self-depreciating humour and Scottish stoicism made him a delight.

It gradually emerged that the great dilemma of his life was that his strong Roman Catholicism made him ashamed of his homosexuality. At the time homosexuality was illegal in Scotland so he had spent a life of isolation. This was determined at the age of nineteen when, after a first, exciting and confirming sexual experience with an older man, Jimmy in a drunken state admitted to his brother that he was gay. The next day, his very Catholic mother banned him from contacting any members of the family until he repented. Jimmy noted that his childhood had been a toxic marinade of rules, guilt, sin and shame.

I made links for him between his childhood, his self-loathing, his isolation and his withdrawal into agoraphobia. We talked about Scottish images of masculinity and how he was an outsider. His agoraphobia seemed an obvious consequence.

Jimmy found our weekly walking sessions more challenging. Close to the clinic where I worked was a very large recreational pond, with a circumference of about five hundred metres. On one side of the pond was a large hotel (called The Pond Hotel - now there's imagination), so I initially invited Jimmy to walk to the hotel and then back on his own. We gradually extended this to him walking past the hotel and around the entire pond.

We then moved to Byres Road, a thriving inner city Glasgow street of shops, restaurants and pubs, plus an underground station. Having mastered navigating the street on his own, I travelled with him on the underground for one stop. Then two, then four, and then he travelled one stop back on his own, and so on.

The treatment plan was text-book. Jimmy grew in confidence. He literally looked better. He stopped having his brother bring him to the clinic and caught a bus. One weekend he decided to travel the entire circular length of the Glasgow metro. He failed to calculate that the metro passed Ibrox Park, home of the Glasgow Rangers football club, and he said the influx of thousands of fans terrified him. But, he coped. He recorded it all in his activity diary that he proudly brought to every session.

We agreed that we would drop our contact to a once a month catch-up talk session. It quickly became clear that, although very enjoyable, they were no longer needed.

At our last session Jimmy asked me to do him a favour. Could I arrange for him to have a tour of the hospital's Alcoholism Treatment Unit? I was surprised and asked him why. He said that he was writing a piece on recovery from alcoholism for a major Scottish newspaper. I duly arranged for him to visit and talk to the staff. The unit's Consultant Psychiatrist also gave freely of his time and, with the current inpatients' agreement, Jimmy even sat in on a group.

Jimmy told me that he had much enjoyed his visit and how friendly everyone was.

Three weeks later, his article appeared in a weekend newspaper. The heading, with his name directly beneath, was "One year sober today!"

He told the story of his treatment. How his psychologist (one Bill Saunders) had, as part of his cure, made him walk past hundreds of pubs and not go in. He talked about how hard it was to walk past, the warmth, the whisky, the comradery, all inside, just there, tantalisingly before his very own eyes; but not for him.

He wrote of walking past four pubs in a row on Byres Road and having the realisation he had never been able to do that before. He talked about travelling on the underground past parts of Glasgow where he used to love to drink. He said how shamed he had been by his drinking and how the psychologist had made it easy for him, by telling him he had agoraphobia not alcoholism. How, for the first time in his life, now a year sober, he felt he belonged.

I was stunned. I realised he must have stopped drinking the day after the registrar and I had seen him at home.

On the following Monday we had the usual ward round. The first case discussed was that of a forty-five-year-old man who had been just been admitted for alcohol dependence. The Charge Nurse said, "Whatever you do don't let Bill see him, he'll think he's an agoraphobic." The room filled with laughter.

Bugger them - psychiatric diagnosis really doesn't matter.

So impossible thing to believe number six: what matters in mental health is never the diagnosis, but only the manner in which you engage with the client.

High quality therapeutic relationships can and do heal the wounds that occur from childhood neglect and abuse. Psychotherapy works. The evidence is that it works irrespective of any given diagnosis. It works because it puts in place a relationship in which the person damaged from childhood neglect and abuse can find solace, understanding, acceptance, curiosity, high levels of regard and most importantly, a space they can trust. You can obviously get the diagnosis totally wrong and still have a successful outcome and this is because, as Dr. Irvin Yalom, has presciently written, "it's the relationship that heals."

So maybe we can have one treatment that works with *all* the 265 putative, socially constructed here today, possibly gone in the next DSM, mental illnesses.

If that is the case, then we only need one diagnosis. That's right - childhood neglect and/or abuse. Or, maybe no diagnosis at all, but just one question: "What Happened To You?"

Chapter Two

What happened to you?

The aetiology of the abnormal can only be understood if what is "normal" is known.

In the critical matter of what causes mental health disorders, it is essential to understand the aetiology of mental wellbeing.

Importantly, research conducted from the 1940s onwards has told us what produces "sane" people. The answer is clear and simple. It is attachment, good attachment. The bedrock of mental wellbeing is to have a "secure base" as a child. The pioneer of this work, John Bowlby, has described how this secure base is realised. It is achieved in multiple, repeated, ordinary, day to day interactions between mother and child. If mum has the capacity to nurture then these interactions gradually develop the child's sense of safety, sense of self, of being lovable and of gradually gaining, from this positive attachment, a sense of being able to emotionally self-regulate and self-soothe.

A positive attachment experience, where the mother is tuned into the child's needs, is also essential for normal brain development.

Allan Schore has written that in providing affective social stimulation, a mother encourages self-regulatory functions with the growth of connections between cortical and subcortical limbic structures. Socialisation experiences in the second year are particularly instrumental for an adaptive cortical system that assists when self-regulating emotional states.

It is contended that it is exactly this learning of the capacity to self-regulate one's emotional state that is critical in the development of good mental health. Clinical experience is that mental "ill health" is predicated on a failure to self-soothe, or to succumb to the sense of being overwhelmed by one's feelings.

Interestingly, Charles Darwin did not say the statement for which he is most famous. He did not write: "It's the survival of the fittest." A rival did.

What Charles Darwin much more usefully stated was:

"It is not the strongest of the species that survives, nor the most intelligent, it is the one most adaptable to change."

The capacity to adapt and change is related to malleability, which is the gift of good nurturance, or, as Louis Cozolini presciently wrote, it is, "The survival of the nurtured."

If you reflect on your childhood friends, how many of them had good secure attachment patterns with their parents?

Additionally, did you have a friend who seemed to be particularly good at self-regulation? That is, they managed their emotions well, did not "lose it" when distressed and were generally able to resist temptation, delay gratification and get on well with everyone. Did they seem to have empathy for others and be slow to criticise or put down anyone?

As it happened, I went to school with AG. His mum was a delight, his dad a very hands-on, funny, dad. AG knew he was loved. They regularly told him so. AG knew he mattered. AG thrived. He was Head Boy at school, gained a scholarship to Cambridge University then did medicine. He married his childhood sweetheart. They had four children all of whom eventually followed him to Cambridge. As a doctor, AG was not only popular with his patients, but with the bureaucracy. He was invited onto various NHS committees and boards. He always ended up being the chairperson. He had the knack of being able to make people get on with each other and somehow he always seemed to get what he wanted. He recently received a knighthood for services to medicine.

Some guys have all the luck.

It is considered that approximately sixty per cent of children have securely attached childhoods and develop as adults with what is known as a "secure attachment" style. Such adults are like AG.

They are :

- compassionate
- slow to anger
- empathetic
- curious about others
- seldom, if ever, censorious or critical
- able to self soothe if they become emotionally distressed.

They also have a good sense of who they are and know they are lovable.

Thus they make secure connections to other people, and fortunately for them, they tend to attract partners who also have secure attachment styles.

Their use of mood-altering substances will be moderate and, unless they encounter a serious, traumatic, life-threatening event, they will not, during their lifetimes, darken the doors of any mental health practitioner.

As the research on attachment came slowly to the fore, evidence of the impact of poor attachment, or adverse childhoods also materialised. The classic, stand out study into the impact of such childhoods occurred almost accidently.

In the mid-1980s, The Kaiser Permanente health facility in San Diego conducted a follow up study of patients who had dropped out of their weight loss program. What surprised the researchers was that the majority of the "drop outs" (some 280 ex-patients) reported that in their childhoods or adolescence, they had been sexually abused. The lead researcher, Dr. Felitti, wondered whether becoming obese was a coping mechanism for the trauma of being sexually abused.

In order to test this hypothesis out, Felitti joined with another researcher, Dr. Robert Anda from the Centre for Disease Control and Prevention, and surveyed over 17,000 Kaiser Permanente members. Although a very skewed sample (seventy-five percent were white, seventy-five percent had college degrees and all had jobs), they were after all members of a health maintenance group - when asked about their childhood experience of nine adverse events, such as sexual abuse, emotional abuse, neglect, violence, mental illness, separation or divorce and parental substance use, twenty-eight percent reported experiencing physical abuse and twenty-one percent sexual abuse.

Importantly, these Adverse Childhood Experiences (ACEs) tended to cluster, with forty percent of this middle class sample reporting two or more adverse experiences, and twelve percent four or more. Significantly, what was pragmatically called a "dose-response" relationship was discovered to exist. The more ACEs participants reported, the greater was the negative impact on their current wellbeing. Interestingly, these negative impacts were both physical and psychological.

In one report, the authors concluded that high-risk health behaviours in adulthood, such as alcohol, drug abuse, smoking, severe obesity and promiscuity, were closely associated with the number of ACEs. This also correlated with ill-health, including cancer, chronic lung disease, heart disease, depression, and a shortened life-span.

Compared to an ACE score of zero, having four Adverse Childhood Experiences was associated with a seven-fold increase in alcohol dependence and six or more Adverse Childhood Experiences was associated with a thirty-fold (3000%) increase in attempted suicide. Even a score of one increases one's susceptibility to anxiety and depression.

(The ACE questionnaire is available at the Harvard University Center on the Developing Child web site).

The implication of this research was clear. The aetiology of mental "illness" lies not in an individual's biology, but in what goes on in their childhood homes.

There is also another very significant issue, which is that the brains of neglected and/or abused children are not the same as those of children who have had positive attachment experiences. Brain scans of neglected and/or abused children show multiple differences from their more fortunate peers.

Importantly, but perhaps not surprisingly, the most significant differences were found in the structural development of regions of the brain that manage emotions and impulse control, as well as how we think about ourselves.

The impact on the brain of Adverse Childhood Experiences have been summarised succinctly by Martin Teicher, a researcher at Harvard University. He noted that the brains of neglected and/or abused children had the following differences:

- the size of the hippocampus is decreased, impacting memory and learning
- there is a decrease in the size of the corpus callosum, whose primary function is to integrate cortical function, i.e. motor, sensory and cognitive function
- the size of the cerebellum is decreased, affecting coordination and motor skills
- a volume decrease in the prefrontal cortex, affecting behaviour, perception and balancing emotions
- high activity in the amygdala, impacting the processing of emotions and reactions to dangerous or stressful situations
- a dysfunctional effect at different levels of hypothalamic-pituitary-adrenal (HPA) axis.

In summary, because of the brain changes brought about by adverse experiences, such children (and adults) are more reactive and are more easily emotionally dysregulated. Or, as Ryan North has very adroitly said,

"Our brains are wired for connection, but trauma rewires them for protection. That's why healthy relationships are difficult for wounded people."

If the above is not persuasive of the corrosive impact that poor childhoods have on mental health, then consider the following.

In the 1980s a team of researchers from Harvard and Duke Universities in the USA evaluated the "levels of maternal warmth" between five hundred mothers and their eight-month-old offspring. The dyads were video taped at Harvard University and then the five hundred tapes were sent to Duke University where the videos were independently evaluated by researchers who specialised in studying attachment. The results of these ratings remained unknown to the Harvard researchers. Then, thirty years later, the Harvard group attempted to contact the five hundred eight-month old babies they had previously videotaped (who were now, of course, all in their early thirties).

Impressively, they managed to follow up 462 of the eight-month-old babies. They got each of these participants to complete the Symptom Check List 90; a standardised screening test of mental health. The SCL 90 assesses nine dimensions of mental health including anxiety, depression, psychosis, hostility, obsessive compulsive behaviour, paranoia and also gives an overall level of distress measure.

Lo and behold, what they found was that those babies who had had "warmer" mothers had significantly fewer mental health issues. The reverse was also true. Low ratings on maternal warmth were associated with higher SCL 90 scores. Significantly, the children of the ten percent of mothers who were worst at being warm, reported exponentially higher levels of mental health symptoms. The authors noted:

"In conclusion, it is striking that a brief observation on the level of maternal warmth in infancy is associated with distress in adult offspring thirty years later. These provocative findings add to the growing evidence that early childhood helps to set the stage for later life experiences, and provides support for the notion that biological "memories" laid down early, may alter psychological and physiological systems and produce latent vulnerabilities or resilience to problems emerging later in adulthood."

Good childhoods donate emotional resilience and vaccinate against madness.

The reverse is also demonstrably true. Poor childhoods cause emotional dysregulation. Poor childhoods disrupt one's capacity to make and hold warm intimate relationships. Poor childhoods make you crazy.

Poor quality childhoods are the true aetiology of all of the putative adult mental health disorders. The aetiology of all of the so-called "mental illnesses" is psychological not biological.

So how was your childhood? How well were you nurtured?

There is an exercise that I use with most of my clients. It is a telling, five question, screening test of this critical issue of "how well-nurtured were you?"

Have a go if you wish, calculate your own score.

Here are the actual, transcripted, responses of one patient, Will, a sixty-five-year-old male. He allowed me to audiotape his responses and use them for teaching purposes.

"Will, I'd like you to think back to the first five years of your life, who was your primary care-giver? Who looked after you most?"

"My mum, definitely my mum, dad was seldom seen."

"Now Will, think back to the first five years of your life. How *Playful* was mum with you? How often did she literally play with you? Things like playing games, having fun at the park, or doing painting and making things? Can you score her on a ten point scale, ten lots, naught none?"

Will hesitated. "Um, I was a twin, my mum had two much older children. My mum was sort of overwhelmed by me and my sister. She was always busy."

I can feel Will defending his mum - a common experience in doing this exercise. We all like to think our parents did their best.

Tellingly, in the Harvard/Duke University study cited above, when the adults were interviewed on follow up, those who had the *least* warm (worst) mothers consistently reported their mums as being average or above average in warmth.

I press Will, "A score out of ten for playfulness?"

A bit more defence. "Eh, look it was post-war England. It was austere."

I wait.

"Okay, no, she wasn't playful at all, hardly ever. I'll give her two, maybe three out of ten."

"Thank you Will, now how about *Love*? How much was it evident to you that your mum loved you? How much could you tell she delighted in you; was besotted by you?"

Will laughs. "Um, I don't think either of my parents did 'besotted' or 'delighted,' just not their thing!"

I nudge Will along, "Okay, score mum out of ten for feeling she loved you, ten lots, naught for none."

Will hesitated. "It's funny, love was never a word that was used in my family. I can remember when I was older, watching a TV show called *The Waltons*, it was an American sitcom. There was a character called 'John boy,' his mum always used to say 'Goodnight John boy, I love you John boy.' It always made me very uncomfortable."

He paused. "Later, when I had my own children, I had to practice saying to them: 'I love you.' I sort of did it indirectly. I used to say it when I put them to bed - 'good night, don't let the beddie bugs bite, see you in the morning, I love you.'"

I nudge him along: "A score out of ten then on the love scale for mum?"

He countered. "Look, I know she loved me, she just never said it."

I wait.

"Oh, okay then, I'll give her a two."

(It's hard to give critical scores to those that we needed nurturance from, especially if we didn't get it).

I go on.

"Now, how about *Acceptance*? How much did mum accept you for being just whom you were, your natural self? Score her out of ten."

For once, Will was onto it straight away. "Oh, that's easy, on a good day one, but usually zero. I always got the message that I was a wimp, that I was a feeble boy, I wasn't up to the mark. Mind you, I was very shy."

"Now Will, how about *Curiosity*? How curious was mum about you, about your development, how intrigued was she with you?"

Will's response is one of bewilderment. "Intrigued? Curious about me? Why, not at all, are mums supposed to be curious about their children?"

I scored that a zero.

Finally, I ask Will about his mother's capacity to empathise with him.

"How good was your mum about being able to see what you were feeling? How good was she at validating your feelings? Letting you know that whatever you were feeling was okay?"

Will reflected. "My mum loved me being happy. If we said we were happy my mum was okay, but every other feeling was not okay. I can remember one day, I was about four, my sister and I were home alone." (Now there's a marker of neglect).

"A gypsy woman knocked on the door trying to sell flowers. My twin sister and I found some coins somewhere and we bought some. I can remember being very upset by the gypsy woman, there was something about her that was desperate. When mum came back I was crying. She said: 'What are you crying about? Stop it.' So, feelings were not really allowed, unless you were happy."

"Will, can you score mum out of ten then for empathy?"

He gave, what I consider is a generous score, of three.

So, on this screening test of "how nurtured were you?" Will scored seven, maybe eight, out of fifty. This is a poor score and was instrumental in understanding his struggles with "depression," with feeling "less than," and drinking excessively.

The majority of my patients score below ten. Not infrequently, people score zero.

My patients have got used to this PLACE analysis. I have unashamedly cribbed it from Dan Hughes, one of the foremost authorities on childhood trauma. He actually uses PACE; he leaves out love. However, I think how loved you felt when you were a child is critical. For me, it is the basis of attachment, but, hey ho, psychologists generally don't agree with each other.

This brings us to the very heart of things. Given that the best predictor of your mental health status as an adult is the quality of your relationship with your primary care giver when you were young, then the focus of our work must shift from the inherently problematic "What's Wrong With You" medical approach to the "What Happened To You?" psychological perspective.

Liz Mullinar is a persuasive champion of this perspective. See https://www.youtube.com/watch?v=svX3fEdVTLQ

As, also, is Dr. Sandra Bloom. Central to her work on the Sanctuary Model is the understanding of the impact of early childhood experience, and diagnosis is absent. Bloom has written that how lovable and worthy we view ourselves to be is determined by our early attachment experiences. These experiences show us how to manage emotions, how to behave and what we expect from others.

Bloom continued to note that parental care, the mother-infant bond, and later the bond between father and infant, is the foundation for all adult bonding, love and friendliness.

Thus, the way ahead is to adopt a model in the management of adults troubled with mental health issues that is based on the premise of a single aetiology, that of childhood neglect and/or abuse, aka, childhood trauma. This concept has been embraced by Bloom in her Sanctuary model and she has articulated an impressive conceptual and clinical perspective that involves clinical agencies adopting, embracing and delivering a totally trauma-informed model.

Unfortunately, there are two related critical impediments to the adoption of such a clever and clinically sophisticated, non-medical model. The first is that most of us work as individuals in essentially "What's Wrong With You?" systems. The second, as only too sadly described by Bloom in her book, *Destroying Sanctuary* is that the very system created to deliver the "What's Wrong With You?" model is under such distress delivering its flawed model that it is incapable of delivering effective services. It is also opposed to change since this would see the end of the medical hegemony in mental health.

This became only too evident to me when, as director and head of psychotherapy at a private psychiatric hospital, my intent to deliver a trauma-based group therapy program was thwarted by the major medical insurer of our clients, who opposed funding of such a group because, "trauma" was not a recognised diagnosis. (PTSD groups could be run, but only for those who had been exposed to single, one-off, life-threatening events).

So we had to run independent "depression", "anxiety" and "addiction" groups. My specific trauma group, known as Strive and Thrive, only came into being because we could "sell" it to the insurance companies as a graduate group for people with "depression", "anxiety" and "drug-dependence."

In 2005, a lead childhood trauma researcher, Dr. Bessell van der Kolk, proposed a new mental health disorder - that of Developmental Trauma Disorder. He noted that children who have been traumatised have a tendency to replicate that trauma in multiple ways in their lives. This manifests in fearful or aggressive behaviour and uncontrolled emotional reactions, as well as avoidance and sexual acting-out.

Despite a plethora of evidence (such as the above studies) and considerable and influential political lobbying, this proposition was not included in DSM

5.0 (2013). It was voted out, not in, despite overwhelming evidence as to its validity.

My suspicion is that the impacts of trauma cut across too many of those reliable and cherished mental illnesses, with their yet-to-be-discovered biological causes.

The epidemiology is that in any month in Australia 18.4% of the population will report having a "mental illness." Interestingly, depression, anxiety and alcohol and drug disorders are the most frequently reported disorders and account for sixty-three percent of the total reported burden of "illness." All of which are, of course, direct consequences of adverse childhood experiences. If one also includes personality disorders (the aetiology of which are officially unknown, but recent research shows that over ninety percent of borderline patients report adverse childhoods), then ninety-two percent of the total burden of so-called "mental illness" can be accounted for by Dr. Bessell van der Kolk's Developmental Trauma Disorder.

If this diagnosis had been allowed in to the good book of DSM 5.0, then it would, in my view, rapidly have become the most commonly diagnosed disorder, and the whole medical, yet-to-be-found-biological-basis of the so-called mental illnesses would have been severely challenged.

In the next chapter, the twenty psychological impacts of childhood trauma are outlined. If these were accepted as being the result of developmental trauma, then again the very basis of DSM 5.0 as it currently stands would be under threat.

In effect, conceptually very different mental "illnesses," for example, depression, anxiety and psychosis, which are all purported to have different biological aetiologies, and therefore require very different psychopharmacological "medicines," would now be seen as having the same non-biological cause.

If such developmental trauma had been included as a discrete disorder in DSM 5.0 or even 5.1, 5.2 or 6.0, then would the grip of psychiatry and the psychopharmacological industry with which it is so closely tied be loosened?

If a developmental trauma perspective were to be introduced, then people with so-called mental illnesses would not be considered ill, not ill at all. They would be seen as reacting to, and living with, the consequences of Adverse Childhood Experiences.

The challenge then would be to introduce effective interventions for children and adults with traumatic childhoods. Such interventions, because the aetiology is psychological, rather than biological, would be psychological.

This is exactly where the "What Happened To You?" field is today. Although there is much dispute as to the optimum psychological intervention for developmental trauma, what is clear is that in the world of therapy, outside psychiatry, the notion of trauma-informed therapy is taking hold.

In the remainder of this book a therapeutic paradigm is outlined via the use of real case studies, of what I consider constitutes trauma informed therapy. Or, perhaps more accurately, therapy that addresses the impacts of "What Happened To You?"

The perspective on trauma that I use in my work is that it comes in two guises, neglect and abuse. Essentially, neglect is parental acts of omission. Neglect is the absence of the right stuff. Abuse is parental acts of commission, the presence of wrong stuff. However, neglect often invites abuse.

Within psychology, there is the persuasion that abuse, be it physical or sexual, is more damaging than neglect. I'm not so sure. One patient, Robyn, once said in group, "It was the grey endless days of neglect that drove me crazy, the abuse not so much."

Robyn's comment made me think that she just may be right.

Over the years, you start to see patients who report that nothing particularly bad, in the form of sexual or physical nastiness, occurred. Yet they present in a flat, often listless manner. When asked, "What brings you to see a psychologist?", they often report being stuck. Stuck in the same boring job, or stuck with no job, stuck in a relationship that they know is unhealthy, or stuck not having a relationship at all. They often engage with therapy very pleasantly, but they stay stuck. Many have been, to absolutely no prevail at all, on "anti-depressants" for years.

My take is that childhood neglect, the grey endless days of it, is managed by children with passivity and withdrawal to an internal world. The trouble is that what keeps you safe as a child is hurtful and harmful in adulthood.

As adults, they do what they did as children. They sit and they watch. And, just as when they were children, they have neither agency nor traction. Agency is having a sense of "I need to go there, do this, be that"; traction is the mojo to put it into action.

The other problem with neglect is that it invites sexual abuse.

David was referred to me by a local GP. The GP said that David was depressed. When I asked him, "What brings you to see a psychologist?" He said, "I'm sort of stuck."

On presentation, David was an affable forty-seven-year-old man who had never married. He worked for a bank as an economist. He said that although he had a PhD in economics, other younger, less well-credentialed people were being promoted over him. He also said that a long term, "on and off again" relationship had finally come to a slithering, dithering halt.

He described living in a four-bedroom house that he had bought a decade previously, because "at the time" he had wanted children. Now he needed to sell it and buy something more suited to his needs, but he just couldn't get around to it.

WHAT HAPPENED?

His story aroused my suspicions. So off to his childhood we went. David said that he was the last of four children. He had three older sisters neatly spaced out in two year intervals ahead of him. He reported that his mother was much consumed by looking after his youngest sister who had cerebral palsy. He always had the impression that his arrival was unintended. "I was a mistake, I was a burden."

He reported that as a child he was often left to his own devices. He recalled many hours as a young child having to entertain himself. He said that he played on his own for hours with his toy soldiers and even made up a test match cricket game that, like the real thing, kept him entertained for days.

As David told of his history, he never mentioned his father. Such lack of comment is always helpful, because it is often the parent that is not talked about who was the most troubling. So I explored this with David.

"Tell me about dad," I said.

His response was quick and to the point. "Never saw him."

"Because?"

"Work, football, womanising, fishing, drinking and golf."

"Ah," I said.

David told me that initially, at primary school, he was quite solitary, struggled to make friends and was, at best, an average student. Then he reported that in the natural progression of moving up a grade at school, a Mr. Webster became his form teacher.

He reported that from the off, Mr. Webster paid him attention. Mr. Webster said that he felt David could do better; that he felt David was underperforming. Mr. Webster gave David a spelling book and asked him to learn eight new words every day. Mr. Webster gave him a times table arithmetic book. David was told "learn five new multiplications every day."

David began to flourish. His English and spelling improved. Arithmetic suddenly became understandable and fun. David reported that by the Christmas of that year he was second in the class. He said that he felt immeasurably better about himself.

David reported that Mr. Webster was also the under-tens football coach and David got into the team. Suddenly, David began to make friends. He said that the highlight of his ninth year was scoring five goals in a game. "Even my father came to watch."

I waited for the inevitable.

David eventually said it. "I was doing so well that Mr. Webster offered to give me extra after class tuition. My mum and dad were very pleased."

"I have never, ever told anyone this, but at the end of every extra tuition session, Mr. Webster would run his hand up my shorts, stick a finger up my arse and have me suck his cock."

Neglect causes abuse. Neglect, the feeling of not being wanted, of being a burden, of not having a sense of being special, makes young people susceptible to the Mr. Websters of the world. David said that although he disliked the sexual activity, when he looked back on his life he knew that without Mr. Webster he would not have got a scholarship to the local, independent, grammar school, would not have gone to university, and would never have achieved a PhD.

Predators like Mr. Webster are adept at spotting isolated, lonely children. Grooming occurs because it is welcomed. Also, predators know that neglected children never tell, because they have no one to confide in.

We agreed that it was his early childhood neglect that left him at forty-seven in limbo. The sexual abuse was yet another consequence of that neglect.

I did not think David was depressed at all. I think he was a victim, and then slowly a survivor, of childhood neglect and abuse.

As a footnote, David slowly found some agency, left the bank he had been at for twenty-five years and is now teaching economics on an MBA course in Sydney. However, he still lives on his own.

I love exploring people's childhoods. I love seeing the implicit messages they have picked up about themselves and how this plays out in their everyday functioning. It is delightful to explore together and determine, "What happened to you to make you be like this?"

"Let's be 'mind detectives' and work out what this is really about."

So, now to the late Dr. Anthony Storr, a British psychiatrist, who wrote what was, for me, the most helpful therapeutic sentence that directly addressed the issue of doing therapy with sometimes very wounded people.

But before we consider that sentence, here is another quote from him that I love. He delightfully wrote about a conversation he had with a director of a monastery. "The director said: 'Everyone who comes to us does so for the wrong reasons.' And I thought the same is generally true for people who become psychotherapists."

Elegantly written by Anthony Stevens, Dr. Storr's obituary was published in the British newspaper, The Guardian. It is a telling piece that sums up the "What Happened To You?" perspective. Although, due to copyright law, I am unable to provide the exact words from that article for you here, I have summarised from the obituary, the details of Storr's life. I think it reflects what I consider to be the zeitgeist of this book.

Storr's work revealed an enduring concern for those trapped in mental suffering, perhaps because of his own experiences with isolation, depression and unhappiness. He held a rich appreciation of the power of self-healing, and was impatient with the clinical model of psychiatry and its symptomatic classification.

WHAT HAPPENED?

His book *The Art of Psychotherapy* was first published in 1979. Not only is it a highly readable text full of wisdom, it also contains that sentence that ought to be taught in every counselling course in the world. In the book, Storr reflects on the nature of psychotherapy, his approach to it, and why psychotherapy works.

Storr wrote that before he saw any new patient he would sit in his room and reflect for a moment on this new encounter. He said that when he stood up and went to open his door he would see written on the door:

"What is it about this patient that I can love?"

Just imagine if you were seeing a therapist and you became aware throughout the sessions that here was someone that you could feel was finding in you something they loved. How would that be?

I believe it is curative. Just as Storr wrote that it changed his life when he thought that CP Snow, his tutor at Cambridge University, liked him, then so for our almost universally not-nurtured-enough clients, feeling loved can be life-changing, even life-saving.

Chapter Three

Dramatic fine spies's

Childhood neglect and trauma have a myriad of negative impacts on adult psychological functioning; understanding and remembering this diversity is difficult. Mnemonic devices are ways of remembering complex things. This chapter is such a device for remembering the array of impacts that follow from childhood neglect and abuse.

Importantly, impacts are not symptoms. This is not a way to diagnose people, but rather a guide to understanding and intervention.

Each of the impacts is treatable. Using this mnemonic device is a way of inviting the patient on a journey of recovery. Working together, you can determine where the focus of the work needs to be done.

The evidence from my practice has been that patients welcomed and appreciated seeing how many impacts they have, and where the main psychological repairs need to be done. There is, however, a "trauma split". Patients demonstrate enormous compassion and acceptance for a fellow traveller, but will hold themselves in high contempt and self-loathing for their own, almost identical, past.

It is fair to say that at the current time (May 2021), there is also a "trauma split" within the field of managing childhood trauma in adults, that is, the field is split on how trauma is best managed.

There are two camps. To be honest, it's more of a chasm than a split!

First, there are those that support and believe that childhood trauma in adults is best managed by *talking* therapies. This can be explored by researching the following therapists: the likes of Judith Beck, Donald Meichenbaum (both cognitive behaviour therapists), Irvin Yalom (existentialist), and Stephen Grosz (psychoanalytical).

On the other side are the *body* therapists. Here reside such luminaries as Pat Ogden, Lisa Schwartz and Peter Levine.

WHAT HAPPENED?

Their basic tenet is that talking therapies are not helpful, and that the way to manage childhood trauma in adults is through specific techniques that allow the body to discharge the stored trauma. It is worth noting that Pat Ogden (sensorimotor psychotherapy), Peter Levine (somatic experiencing), and Lisa Schwartz (Comprehensive Resource Model) are all charismatic therapists who have, from their clinical experience, developed their own models of intervention. This is practice-based evidence at work.

The problem is that each firmly believes that their way is best, but all are united against the talking therapy fraternity. It can get very tense.

Take, for example, the matter of Eye Movement Desensitisation and Reprocessing (EMDR). Brought into clinical practice by Francine Shapiro, EMDR is demonstrably effective in treating trauma of the one-off life-threatening event kind. Essentially, anyone who personally experiences, or witnesses such an event can be susceptible to what is now known as Post Traumatic Stress Disorder (PTSD).

Trauma, from the Greek word for hurt, occurs when a person experiences an event that is outside the range of usual human experience. The impact of such an event is subjective. Because of their childhood's, people have different capacities or resilience to managing distress. The key is how threatened and helpless they felt during the life threatening event. In effect, had the person's coping mechanism been overwhelmed?

In EMDR, the therapist uses their fingers to create a flicker-like motion in front of the patient's eyes. Although this sounds strange, this therapy has been shown to significantly reduce a patient's PTSD.

However, not everyone agrees. Meichenbaum, for example, has adroitly reflected his disdain for such methods by saying, "I give the finger to the fingers." Such is the tension in the managing trauma field.

Given where we are at the present time, my belief is that anyone entering the field of counselling would be wise to undertake training that is offered by the various *body* schools of trauma management. It is my firm belief that the future of treating trauma will be the "What Happened To You?" perspective rather than the "What's Wrong With You?" medical model.

Despite my affirmation in the above paragraph, this book embraces a combination of *both body and talking* therapies. And because of my training and experience, I'm actually more comfortable with talking than body work, thus the clinical work described throughout the book has a foundation of talking therapy, with a dash of body work techniques.

Getting back to the impact of childhood trauma, what does a childhood of adverse experiences of developmental trauma do to you?

Outlined below are twenty of the most common and most frequently reported psychological impacts of an adverse childhood.

The mnemonic device to assist you in recalling these impacts is:
DRAMATIC FINE SPIES'S

D is for Dissociation

Briefly, dissociation is absence, a disappearing. This can occur gradually, but for most traumatised patients, they will be with you one moment, and gone the next. Dissociation is the brain's protective device. It removes the patient from a perceived situation of threat. A telling sign that patients have the capacity to dissociate is for them to report that, for example, when driving they get lost, and suddenly come to miles from where they were going. Another is that they lose time. As an example, they will report, being at home doing something, and then, in no time at all, it is two hours later.

There is another important clinical matter. Patients' susceptibility to "disappear" will change. They may, for a period of time, be quite present. However, if a patient complains that they are "losing time" or that they are becoming increasing vague, bear with them. In all probability, what is happening is that a repressed memory of something terrible that happened to them is coming back into consciousness. Increased levels of dissociation are a good marker that something dark is coming to light. Especially in the body therapy schools, there are new ways of managing dissociation.

Another clinical trick is to introduce the patient to the notion of "fuzzy." Having a patient indicate by words or a hand signal that they are going "fuzzy" is a good indicator of "ah, we are onto something." You can then work together as mind detectives to determine what had been touched on that caused the "fuzziness."

It is important to stress to patients that dissociation is a protective device that is a normal part of human experience.

R is for Relational intensity

For some patients, their significant relationship becomes literally a matter of life and death. The need for the other is so strong that any hint of instability, of "not being seen," or of "not mattering" to the other prompts acute distress. A key factor in young male suicides is the loss of a girlfriend and many female overdoses are triggered by a break-up. The urgency to be in or have a relationship in some clients is palpable. It often goes like this report from one client: "I cannot be alone, because that tells me I am unlovable, which is unbearable, but being in a relationship is torture, because at any moment it could end. It's exhausting."

A is for Abandonment issues

According to Irvin Yalom, there are three universal concerns about intimacy. The first is that "I will be abandoned," the second is that "I will be colonised" (turned into a mini version of the other), and the third is that "I will be exploited."

For traumatised patients, the key issue is usually abandonment. Neglect especially inculcates a message of "I'm not lovable," so being in a relationship becomes very challenging. In terms of attachment theory, such patients have a "disorganised" attachment style, or in non-formal terms such people are "clingers."

Funnily enough, we tend to look out or scan for whichever of the three great concerns about intimacy that we have. If, for example, you have grown up with three big sisters, a mother and grandmother, then you will know all about being colonised. So in your adult relationship you will react poorly to your partner imposing her guidance over, say, your choice of socks. Those with a childhood in which there were consistent messages of being unlovable will read between the lines and see markers of lack of love everywhere, and those of an exploitation bent will be able to spot being "taken advantage of," or "being used" at a thousand yards. The intensity of this can be remarkable.

I was once seeing a very stylish couple. Both were in their thirties, he was a successful architect and she, after a modelling career, opened a very profitable dress boutique. After having seen them on four or five occasions the following occurred.

She arrived at my office for their next appointment in a fury. She was on her own. Now a couple is a couple is a couple. Her fury needed to be managed, but between the three of us. I was told Derek was coming, and that he was a bastard. A few minutes, later a sheepish, dishevelled Derek arrived. I opened the session with, "I can see that Mary is very upset, so what's on your agenda today?"

Mary launched into it. "He's a fucker, he doesn't love me."

Derek, in classic male logic mode, said something unhelpful like, "But, babe I do!"

"No, you don't, you bastard, after what you did, you clearly don't!"

The secret here is to hear the story.

"Mary, Derek doesn't love you because?"

"Because we'd just had sex, we've been getting on much better of late and I realised that we needed to get a move on to get here on time. So, I asked Derek to make me some tea while I hurriedly showered."

"Which I did!" said Derek defending himself. (Shut up, Derek, and listen).

Mary glared at him, "And then, as I was drying my hair, I asked him to make me some toast and jam. He doesn't fucking love me!"

"Because?"

"Because, when he gave me the toast he had just lumped some butter on the middle of the toast and then just dumped some strawberry jam on top of the unmelted butter."

Ah, gotcha Mary.

So I said, "People who love you, Mary, would spread out the butter, let it melt, and then spread out the jam smoothly to the edges."

"Yes," says Mary triumphantly to Derek, "Bill knows what love is!"

Ah well, not quite. What I know is that love is how you experienced love when you were a child.

What I certainly know is that people who have abandonment issues will scan for any indication that they are about to be abandoned.

Given the improvement in their relationship, Mary's radar for rejection was on very high gain, looking for what she didn't want to see - any sign that her re-established sense of attachment with Derek (that she desperately craved) was about to be rent asunder.

When it comes to attachment and fears of intimacy, we are often our own worst enemies. In unpacking what had occurred, Derek and I learned that Mary's mother, a distant and depressed woman, with whom it was very hard to connect, would on occasions offer a tiny glimpse of warmth by making Mary careful obsessional meals, including immaculate jam on toast for breakfast.

M is for Mood instability

One impact of having a traumatising childhood is that, in adulthood, your moods can change frequently, happy one moment then sad, then angry, back to content, and then a march into rage.

It is exhausting having such precarious moods. This of course invites the prescription of heavy duty so-called "mood stabilisers" that actually are either anti-epilepsy drugs or "anti-psychotics." Your moods are stabilised by having a handbrake applied to your brain. This is of limited palliative use and no lasting therapeutic value.

The solution with mood instability is to explore the triggers of such volatility and attempt to identify what is occurring. Knowing the latent causes of why your mood plunges or soars is an essential part of re-gaining balance. Understanding your moods, rather than controlling or dampening them down, allows the eventual use of self-soothing techniques. Such techniques include breathing, meditation, mindfulness, yoga - and the best is talking. Learning that when distressed having someone to talk to and be with you, is literally the best medicine, is often a surprise and a shock to those of us whose childhoods lacked such solace. Learning that emotional distress is manageable, that emotional dysregulation need not be overwhelming, is the ultimate cure for childhood trauma.

A is for Anger (aka rage)

Anger is a universal emotion. We all have the capacity to get angry. However, childhood trauma breeds rage, the hurricane equivalent to the storm of anger. Rage is destructive, and not just to the object of one's rage, but also to the self. For some people, their rage comes on so fast that it not only seems unmanageable, it also seems unpredictable and frightening. Some patients believe that their rage is a marker of their craziness. Yet anger is, as outlined in a subsequent chapter, merely an acute, wired-in, reptilian brain response, to a perceived threat. So rage is best managed by understanding the childhood wound that gets triggered, and what "hurt" it is that causes you to explode.

T is for Trust

Trust comes in different guises. For, example do you trust your partner with your money? Do you trust them with your possessions? Do you trust that you are physically safe with them? Do you trust them sexually? Do you trust them emotionally?

It is the last question that is the most tricky for many traumatised patients. Being emotionally vulnerable is, if you were neglected and or abused as a kid, very dangerous, almost impossible. Imagine if as young boy, you were constantly bullied by your three older brothers, physically abused by your father and ignored by your mother. Imagine being tied up and staked out on the ground by your brothers and then being left in a paddock to the mercy of the weather, ants, insects and possibly snakes. Imagine that your brothers would return some time later and encourage cattle to defecate on you. Imagine, when tied up and helpless your brothers, would themselves urinate and defecate on you. Imagine your powerlessness, your rage as you laid out there, sometimes in blistering heat or storms, just having to wait for your release, especially knowing that your parents were disinterested as to your whereabouts.

When Adam, a sixty-year-old-man told me the above about his childhood, I was impressed he could even sit in the room with me and trust me to listen.

What I loved about Adam was his self-reliance, his understanding that trauma had made him different from other non-traumatised people, his vulnerability, and that he was still alive. He still hoped that his life would improve.

After a year of regular trauma informed psychotherapy he actually allowed me to give him a hug. We both had tears in our eyes.

C is for Chronicity

One of the most painful impacts of trauma is that it sticks with you. The impacts become familiar, but such a familiarly is draining, exhausting, and perpetual. It colours your world. I always explain to "What Happened To You?" patients, that their childhoods were not like other peoples.

Believe it or not, I say, about sixty per cent of children have good childhoods; they have childhoods that rate from thirty to fifty on the PLACE scale. They have secure attachment styles. They seldom, unless some very nasty life event occurs, such as the loss of a child or partner, come into therapy.

However, I say to the survivors of childhood neglect and abuse, you are not like them. You do not have a secure attachment style. You will have most, if not all, of the impacts of neglect and abuse. You will be a DRAMATIC FINE SPIES's type of person. You will not be like the normal people who had lovely childhoods, so please stop trying to be normal.

In Elizabeth Strout's painful book entitled *My name is Lucy Barton*, she writes this in the character of Lucy:

"... when I see others walking with confidence down the sidewalk, as though they are completely free from terror, I realise I don't know how others are."

As so elegantly expressed above, neglect and/or abuse in childhood makes one different, makes one's world different.

The first step in this type of therapy is to nudge the client into some acceptance that what most unfairly happened to them, did actually happen. Then the task is to work together to reduce, modify, and manage those impacts.

I always say, "You are totally normal; normal for someone who has been neglected and abused. But striving to be like the normal, well-attached, nice childhood people, will only exhaust you."

F is for Flashbacks

Flashbacks are visual images of past trauma. They can be very disturbing and have an eerily obtuse presentation. Some will be like fragments of a past event a snippet here and there; a video that has been chopped up and then randomly re-assembled. Careless or uninformed clinicians can mistake flashbacks as being psychotic symptomatology. One patient of mine, who had been tied up and sexually abused by the son of friends of the family, was prescribed anti-psychotics because she complained of seeing things. What she was seeing was visual snippets of her repetitive rapes.

If you have ever been in a serious road traffic accident, something unusual may have occurred just prior to the collision. Many people report that just prior to an accident, when they knew it was inevitable, everything went into slow motion. Familiar?

WHAT HAPPENED?

This is because your brain, sensing danger, tips adrenalin, cortisol and other "make-your-brain-go-faster-in-order-to-escape" chemicals into your brain. As your brain goes into overdrive, your logical brain lags behind. So your visual world slows down.

There is another problem. How we remember things is a three phrased system. First, if something new comes into view, you will "encode it" for future use; like taking a snapshot. This is then passed into phase two, which is our short-term memory. This snapshot is held in your short-term memory for about ten to twelve seconds, when it is then passed into long-term memory where it can be stored. Each memory is than tagged with various tentacles so that later it can be recalled.

Imagine that you are driving rather fast. You notice in your rear view mirror that there is a white car, with blue and red lights on its roof, and bright visible stripes down the sides. Yes, it's a police car! You were able to retrieve that initial snapshot of a police car without wasting time thinking, "oh what's that?" Hopefully, this encoded and instantly retrieved information, avoided you getting a fine.

For those of you of British extraction, think of a Panda car. Bing, it's in your brain. Whereas Australians may have pictures in their heads of cuddly animals with black eyes, the Brits will be recalling the strange obsession every British police force had in the 1970-80s of buying very ordinary cars, painting them light blue-green and white and driving around in what were known as Panda cars.

But, here is a real problem. If your brain is tripped into emergency mode, that very activation will sever the link between your short-term and your long-term memory. Thus you will, after you have (hopefully) survived that road traffic accident, have to manage your brain trying to recover the bits of visual and auditory memory that never found its proper storage place in your long-term memory system. Thus, flashbacks are not a psychotic symptoms, it is just your brain trying to recover unsorted, un-stored memories.

There is an expression in the therapeutic management of flashbacks, and its two associated markers that are coming up next, which is important.

It is, "In order to forget you have to remember."

Patients who have survived serious assaults, vicious rapes or attempts to murder them frequently have flashbacks, intrusive thoughts and nightmares. Although they can be terrifying, it is normal. It's the brain trying its hardest to remember what happened. The trick of this is to help the person recall what occurred so that they can store the fragmented bits of memory in their long- term memory. Once in long-term memory it can, like all memories, be forgotten. Thus, "In order to forget you have to remember."

I encourage patients to play flashbacks like a video on to a handy blank wall.

Go towards your flashbacks, not away from them. Bring them on, get them out in the open, put them where they belong, in your long-term memory - and then you can forget them.

I is for Intrusive thoughts

As with flashbacks, intrusive thoughts can have a nasty horrible impact. Things you don't want to remember just pop into your head. This has been most precisely described by Lucy Barton who noted, "This must be the way that most of us manoeuvre through the world, half knowing, half not, visited by memories that can't possibly be true."

N is for Nightmares

This third feature of the brain trying to forget is often the most alarming. Patients will become terrified to fall asleep, and may use heavy doses of alcohol or benzodiazepines to block the nightmares out. Some doctors have tried prescribing beta-blockers to slow down your heart rate so you don't wake up, but all the avoidance tactics are, in my view, an error.

Again, I think nightmares need to be approached from the perspective of "what is this nightmare telling me that I had not recalled in the past?" I recommend a notebook by the bed, and the use, on awakening terrified, of various types of breathing to calm your terrified nervous system.

Adam, from above, was a case in point. Although very reluctant, he took on board my salutation to go toward his flashbacks, develop his intrusive thoughts, and "delight" in the valuable information his nightmares were telling him. Over the course of a year, they diminished to becoming a rarity. (Albeit, if he got anxious about something else in his life, then that heightened arousal did bring them back). However, yoga, meditation, mindfulness and breathing can all help. Whereas beta-blockers, alcohol, benzodiazepines and "anti-psychotics" will all just prolong the agony.

So, remember, "In order to forget you have to remember."

E is for Emotional dysregulation

Emotional dysregulation is a hallmark feature of childhood neglect and abuse, and probably is the most distressing. Emotional dysregulation is being distressed by your own distress. Literally you become afraid, terrified, of your own feelings; feelings that are overwhelming and unmanageable. This is a re-enactment of what occurred in the past when there was no one there for you.

I have an exercise that you may wish to try.

Imagine that you are eight years old again. You have had a bad day at school.

WHAT HAPPENED?

You may have been bullied, chastised unfairly, had to read something out, made a mess of it and everyone laughed at you. Whatever it was, imagine that you are now leaving school at the end of the day. You are very heavy hearted.

You arrive home; what would you have done next?

Interestingly, whenever I use this exercise with clients, I get the following type of answers.

"Oh, I'd go to my room," "I'd go down the park and hide there," "I'd just go off on my own," "I'd go for a bike ride," "I'd go out and play with my mates," "I'd eat cake," "I'd beat up my younger brother."

I seldom get, "Oh, I'd go home and talk to mum about it, she'd make me feel better."

If I do get "I'd go tell mum about it," it usually comes with a qualifier, like "I'd tell mum, but she'd just overreact and storm off to the school," or "I'd tell mum and she'd get angry," or "I'd try and tell mum, but she wouldn't listen."

Well, how did you go?

The secret to emotional regulation is to have had a primary care giver who, when you were small and hurt, listened. As noted above, emotional dysregulation is caused by neglect and abuse, by having no one who, when you were hurt, stopped and listened. Intimacy has been defined as "when you hurt, my world stops, and I listen." That is, of course, a completely novel idea for adults with adverse childhood experiences.

Interestingly, I have a follow-up question. When in group I say, "Now how many of you still do the same thing?"

It takes a moment, but those dependent on alcohol or other substances say "Yes, I still go off on my own." Others will acknowledge that when emotionally hurt they isolate themselves; others literally distract themselves by exercise or eating, or by violence, just as they did when they were young.

Our response to emotional distress is laid down by the time we are eight. It often takes careful psychotherapy to enable people to give up the defences of their childhood. Defences that worked as a child become hurtful and harmful as an adult. It is often very hard to do "emotional distress" differently.

The trick of emotional distress is to literally be able to sit with your distress and self-soothe. Self-soothe by talking, by being vulnerable, by being open, by being intimate, by breathing, by meditating, by mindfulness. But, not by using substances, acting out or in, by self-harming or raging.

Here's a funny thing. There's a trick or two of being able to soothe really emotionally distressed people. One is just sit and be with them. If they allow just touch their hand, or less intrusively, place your foot on their foot (with shoes on!)

The other is this. One evening, I was walking out of my office that at the time was adjacent to a psychiatric ward. As I walked through the adjoining garden

I heard a commotion. I went to investigate and discovered a very angry young female patient screaming at a formidable male nurse.

I sensed that the patient was tipping into violence, so I placed myself between the protagonists and said to the petite patient, "I can see you are very angry."

"Fuck you!" she said.

"When you are this angry, what do you need?"

"I need my fucking bong back!" (Ah, I now understand what's going on).

I said, "I get it, but when you are this angry what do you need emotionally?"

The young patient looked at me. She was bewildered.

"Need? Emotionally? Fucked if I know."

"Yes, that's the problem, isn't it? You're feeling overwhelmed and you literally don't know how to fix it."

She burst into tears. The formidable nurse retreated, I sat with the patient for a while and calm was restored. (She never got her bong back).

Try it.

1. "When you feel like this, what do you need?" (You will get a logical answer).

2. "When you feel like this, what do you need emotionally?"

You will get an emotional answer like, "I need comfort," "I need understanding," or "I don't know."

Sadly, the most traumatised patients are the most emotionally dysregulated patients, and they have no idea what they need emotionally.

The purpose of good psychotherapy is to show them. They need connection, they need to talk, they need intimacy, they need to be vulnerable, and they need to trust. They need to be seen, heard and held; they need some of Anthony Storr's love.

S is for Self-harm

Whenever I see a patient who has multiple scars on his or her arms or body from cutting themselves, I look directly at their scars and I say, "Congratulations on your survival."

This recognition that cutting is a way of coping always strikes a chord. Patients usually say thank you. It's a thank you for understanding.

I get really irritated when the words self-harm and suicide are used as synonyms. They are not. Cutting is a way of coping (with acute emotional dysregulation); suicide is a way of dying. They are absolutely not the same.

When someone cuts or burns themselves or punches walls, they are inciting pain. Pain turns off your brain because the threat it was preparing you for has now occurred. Cutting, burning, punching holes in walls, work. People who self-harm are not wishing to die, they are wanting to live, but without the distress that they do not know how to manage.

The solution is not a telling off or threats of discharge(!) but an invitation that connection, not cutting, is a better solution. "When you feel like this, what do you need emotionally?" opens a channel of connection that resolves self-harm, usually quickly.

P is for Psychosis

The link between childhood neglect and/or abuse and psychosis is disputed. Yet the evidence that psychosis is a consequence of childhood neglect and abuse is, in fact, very robust. Consider this.

Research teams at Liverpool University and Maastricht University in the Netherlands, analysed findings from over thirty years of studies into childhood trauma and psychosis. Data from more than 27,000 research papers was considered, from three types of studies; research on psychotic patients who were questioned about their early years, studies addressing children known to have childhood trauma, and general research into randomly selected groups.

Results of all the studies led to a similar conclusion. Children with a traumatic experience prior to the age of sixteen, were three times more likely to experience psychosis as adults, as compared to the randomly selected population. A link was found between the level of trauma, and the likelihood of experiencing mental illness later in life. Children who were severely traumatised were at a higher risk, sometimes up to fifty times increased, compared to those who experienced lesser or no trauma.

The team from Liverpool University conducted a new study, looking at the type of trauma experienced, and specific psychotic symptoms. Hallucinations, were associated with sexual abuse, for example, while paranoia was common among those brought up in a children's home.

Why people who have been sexually abused subsequently experience hallucinations, is up for debate, and in terms of the aetiology of schizophrenia, it is a very important debate to develop further. Although totally rejected by mainstream psychiatry as a heresy, the concept that schizophrenia can be caused by childhood abuse has been proved to be true. Well, at least sufficiently for a judge in a British court.

The British Medical Journal in 2007 cited a case in Birmingham, UK, where a man in his thirties was awarded a large sum of money as the judge accepted the claimant was suffering schizophrenia caused by his childhood sexual abuse by a Catholic priest.

Clinical experience shows that paranoia is also a very common consequence of childhood abuse. This process is easy to comprehend, especially if you have been neglected or abused by someone who was supposed to love you. Thus, the very person who thought you could trust, you couldn't. The trouble with such betrayal is it makes you doubt yourself. If you can't trust those who love you, who can you trust? Also, is it your fault? Is your trust radar giving you false information? Can you trust your sense of who you can trust?

Then, if your overall level of distress is ratcheted up a notch or two by having, say, an argument with a partner or parent, or losing a job, or having to move, or being financially even worse off than normal, then this elevation in your emotional level will inevitably rack up your scanning of the world.

As you feel more threatened, then you really need to have good information coming in about your safety. However, as the sense of threat increases, your doubts about your ability to reliably scan those that are safe, from those that are not, increases. So the solution to this is to be hypervigilant, hyper-suspicious. So you re-double your efforts.

Safety can be achieved by monitoring your phone more carefully, placing extra locks on your doors and windows, not going outside, or only going out at night. Then with your heightened suspicion, you may just hear the doorbell ring, but no one is there. You may hear a thud, but no obvious cause. Your phone may ping, but there is no message. There may be people whispering in the garden, but no one is there. However, paranoia is.

Interestingly, when running groups I sometimes, irrespective of the actual topic, say, "Hey guys, how many of you have experienced weird stuff?"

This question always prompts two responses. The first, a bemused "What do you mean?" The second, "Oh yeah."

The "what do you mean?" people have never had any whiff of psychosis, whereas the "oh yeahs" will report having heard something that didn't make sense, or having seen things that couldn't be true? Or, believed things that they later go, "Ah, that was crazy!"

In any group, be it for depression, anxiety, trauma, alcohol and drug dependence, about sixty percent of the participants will somewhat ruefully say ,yes, they have experienced weird stuff. When I explore with them what was happening for them at that time, the overwhelming answer is that they were unusually anxious or distressed, thus their protective radar was scanning at its highest level. The trouble is the harder you look, the easier it is to find … something sinister.

My response to everyone who is exhibiting the tentacles of paranoia, hallucinating, or believing weird things to be true, is to encourage them to live lives of enormous boredom. Just for now, live life at ten percent.

I invite them to hibernate, to withdraw and embrace solitude; to avoid people and places that concern them, to literally give themselves a break. I suggest if they can manage it, some yoga or mediation, maybe in a group, but certainly on their own. I invite them to remember different ways of breathing, or practice mindfulness, be in the now, be gentle with themselves, and that this too will pass. As their anxiety comes down, so will their psychosis. I also invite them to talk to someone they trust about the weird stuff.

I is for Intoxication and Impulsivity

These two "I"s are separate, but linked. Many people who have been neglected and/or abused as children use substances to soothe. In a way, like self-harm, becoming intoxicated with any drug is soothing in that it can relieve, for now, your distress. Unfortunately, the next day your distress has usually returned, often with reinforcements that can prompt another bout of intoxication.

Winston Churchill is credited with saying, "The only proper intoxication is conversation," but I doubt he was really presciently proposing talking as a way out of distress. From attending his museum in London, he clearly relied on alcohol intoxication to regularly soothe his demons.

Many adults traumatised as children can be bewildered by their impulsivity, which if impulsive enough, can invite the label of "bipolar." This impulsivity can be about buying, spending, having sex, drinking, collecting or travelling. If you ask traumatised adults, they will often tell you of outrageous, reckless things they have done on the spur of the moment.

One patient saw an attractive stranger standing at a bar, walked up to him and invited him outside for sex, and got arrested in the process of carrying out her impulsivity. Another bought forty-two pictures at an auction and a day later hated all of them. A third managed to buy two Rolls Royces, in the same afternoon, that he really did not need. Another bought 250,000 shares at a "bargain price" that eventually caused him to file for bankruptcy. As a final example, one very reserved, sober accountant went to his local airport, took the first flight he could get on, and ended up eight hours later in Dubai, where he stayed for a month and co-habitated with a local sex worker.

All of the above were impulsive attempts to literally get away from themselves, to bring some distance to their own distress, some escape from their self-loathing, but unfortunately, in time, such impulsive efforts just added to it.

There is also a significant issue here that often goes undetected. Many traumatised adults are prescribed "anti-depressants." There have been many clinical reports that the long-term use of "anti-depressants" can cause people to become so serene that they become disinhibited.

I once did a court report about a charming seventy-two-year-old retired civil servant, with a totally unblemished past, who had been arrested for stealing some twenty sets of underwear that, she exclaimed to me, were "to die for" and that her husband would "really appreciate." She was unperturbed about her offending.

Following an MRI brain scan (normal) psychometric testing (normal), her GP perceptively took her off her "anti-depressant," prescribed some two years earlier to manage her anxiety. A month or so later, in a follow-up interview, I was confronted by a contrite and concerned offender.

E is for Empty

Particularly when working with women who have been neglected and/or abused as children you will run into the refrain, "I don't know who I am!" They will refer to a constant and nagging sense of being empty. Unsure of their identity they can often report being chameleons, flitting into and out of roles that the background of their lives invite.

This sense of "empty" is often reflected in their sexual behaviour. Many will report using sex as a way to get attention, to get connection, but as one patient frustratedly told me about herself, "Why do I think my value is in my vagina and not in me?"

Not a hard question to answer, as she had been sexually abused by her stepfather from an early age. She had been implicitly told she was valuable as a sexual object, but not as a young girl. Her mother's refusal to believe her, needing the relationship with her new husband more than that with her, also implied "I don't value you, you are not a priority."

The patient in question also lamented that when she got into a relationship she could not shift from sexual object to sexual subject, i.e., be connected and loving. She articulately put her finger right on the issue when she said, "I can fuck, but I can't make love."

If your early sexual experiences are of being "done to," it's very difficult to then shift to "being with" a sexual partner.

The solution to feeling empty, albeit a slow and gradual one, is to be felt. The process of psychotherapy is one that can give empty a sense of substance. The connection, being seen, being heard, being tuned into, being well-regarded, experiencing being enough, being taken seriously, mattering and being held, and yes, loved, are all restorative.

Yet again, "it's the relationship that heals."

S is for Shame

People often confuse guilt with shame. I am not sure why, as they are distinctly different.

Guilt is about things I do; shame is about who I am.

Guilt is not a universal emotion, not everyone has it. Shame is. Everyone can feel shame, and of all the universal emotions, shame is the one that my clinical practice has told me is the most distressing and troublesome.

Shame is about who I am:
- "I am not enough"
- "I don't matter"
- "I'm stupid"
- "I'm weak"
- "I'm vulnerable"
- "I'm powerless"
- "I'm ugly"
- "I'm irrelevant"
- "I'm useless"
- "I'm helpless"
- "I'm unlovable"
- "I'm too much"
- "I'm wrong"
- "I'm dumb"
- "I'm dishonourable"
- "I'm defective"
- "I'm at fault"
- "I'm a mess"
- "I'm a fuck up"
- … and even "I'm a crazy cunt."

These perceptions of self are totally corrosive, they are toxic, but they are not our fault. Shame is inculcated into you by your childhood experiences of your value. Yes, we all have the capacity for shame, but only some of us have been rendered undone by it. Shame is engendered by neglect. Neglect tells us we are not worthwhile. As noted above, neglect changes the way our brains work. Shame is also caused by the acts of another.

As Augusten Burroughs has so perceptively written about shame:

"Shame is a landfill emotion. It's not organic, like joy. It was dumped there by somebody else."

And … "Inside of disappoint is a deeper judgement: less than inferior, defective. Shame can lead to a shitload of problems."

When working in a group when shame is being addressed, I ask each participant to stand up and tell the group of the less good aspects of their natures. Everyone can do that with ease. The room is rapidly overloaded with self-loathing and self-criticism.

I then flip the coin over. What are the best aspects of their natures? Hardly a word is said. If words are said they are said haltingly, without conviction.

Then I invite each participant to write down something they love about each of the other participants. Each member then gets notes saying what it is other people love about them.

I then invite the group to discuss why they do not believe what is written on their notes. They never do. But the realisation that being praised is inimical and self-loathing automatic brings an awareness of their trauma-induced distortion.

However, shame is an emotion, so logic is never enough to shift it. There is after that exercise always a comment by one or other of the group members which is, "Yeah, yeah I know this in my head, but I don't feel it."

Absolutely shifting from self-loathing to self-acceptance, from self-criticism to self-compassion, is a long journey. But, as related in a later chapter, it can be done.

S is for Suicidal ideation and/or action

There is a very useful suicide screening test. It is the Kessler K-10. You can find it online (www.beyondblue.org.au).

Essentially, you fill in ten questions that look to be about anxiety and depression from the perspective of how you have been feeling over the past thirty days. However, the Kessler scale is a scale about psychological distress, which in my view, is a more useful perspective than the categorical anxiety and depression labels.

My clinical experience in using this scale with hundreds of clients is that it is a very valuable screening tool. Screening tests sort out those who probably do versus those that probably don't have condition X or Y. There is with the online version of the K-10 an official scoring criteria, but it unfortunately, having labelled itself a distress measure, then talks in terms of the probability of any score being indicative of the respondent having a mental health disorder. I prefer to sit with levels of distress, because it fits with the patients' personal experience and has a certain "in vivo" validity.

My informal scoring system is: ten to twenty represents low, normal levels of distress. In clinical practice you will only see this type of score toward the end of successful interventions. Twenty to thirty are the usual intake psychological distress scores, but that is obviously influenced by where you work and your case load.

Thirty to forty are indicative of significant levels of psychological distress that may merit, if it has not already occurred, the use of a short term prescription of an "anti-depressant." Obviously this needs to be discussed with the client and his/her GP or psychiatrist.

However, scores above forty are of concern. The evidence is that suicidality, (thinking about, really thinking about, being attracted to and attempting to end one's life), increases exponentially with every increment in scores above forty.

For the clients scoring forty and over, my practice has always been to involve a medical practitioner and a family member in the patient's on-going management. Suicide, its management and prevention, is more fully explored in chapter nine.

So, the above are the twenty consequences or impacts of having a childhood in which there was either not enough of the right stuff and/or too much of the wrong stuff, or both.

As a footnote, I used to put these impacts up on a whiteboard when running what were officially labelled "anxiety" groups. Most of the participants would acknowledge "having" most of them.

I used to also list them on a whiteboard when running "addictions" groups, and most participants had most of them.

Likewise, in so-called "depression" groups, most participants had most of them.

And, of course, in "trauma" groups, almost all of the participants had all of them.

Most tellingly, when I was involved in running groups for people with so-called Borderline Personality Disorder, all the participants scored almost all of them.

Borderline Personality Disorder is the diagnosis that no one wants. Initially, the term borderline was meant kindly. Borderline patients were deemed not to fit in the neurotic/psychotic dichotomy. Borderline patients literally were a bit of both, but not enough to fit in either. They were thus in between or on the borderline. However, the term borderline has become a pejorative term that no one wants.

The important thing about Borderline Personality Disorder is, as Judith Herman so presciently described in 1992, and others such as Marsha Linehan have further refined, Borderline Personality Disorder is not a disorder of personality at all.

It is the direct consequence of being traumatised as a child. Ninety percent of so-called borderline patients give clear histories of childhood trauma involving both neglect and sexual or physical abuse. My perspective is that the remaining ten per cent have either been so traumatised that they have tightly repressed it, or they were victims of neglect that was so pervasive that they just accepted it as normal.

Perhaps for those of us in the "What Happened To You?" camp, maybe the next big political challenge is to make the DSM 5.1 or 5.2, or even 6.0, committee to reverse their decision to reject childhood trauma as a diagnostic category. If homosexuality can be removed by activists, if PTSD can be put in due to the work of combat veterans, then maybe childhood trauma activists can demand and force childhood trauma into the psychiatric bible.

Or, then again, maybe we'll just leave psychiatry on its own with its increasing untenable "What's Wrong with You?" perspective.

There is another reason for leaving psychiatry out. In the UK's National Institute for Clinical Excellence (NICE) clinical guidelines for the management of so-called Borderline Personality Disorder, they found that no form of psychopharmacology had been found to be of clinical value.

Irrespective of which, the Australian evidence is that most "borderline" patients will be on three different types of psychiatric medication; namely an "anti-depressant", an "anti-psychotic" or a "mood-stabiliser."

It is also relevant to note that recent research into personality disorders questions the thirteen or so explicit entities that make up the personality disorders. Indeed, what seems to be going on is that twelve of them are merely variations on a major theme; that of Borderline Personality Disorder; that of developmental trauma.

Thus, all the definite, robust, reliable, valid, personality disorders outlined in the DSMs, are in all probability just variations of the differential impact of childhood neglect and abuse.

The following chapters are case studies of real people with real impacts from childhood neglect and abuse. In order to maintain confidentiality I have changed names, sometimes countries, sometimes made subtle obscuring differences in occupation or ages. However, each case history is true. Where there is dialogue, it is of course a fiction, but a fiction driven by how I work, and what I know I would have said, and what I recall people said. Some of the histories reported are shocking and unbelievable, but they are all true. They are presented in no particular order, but I have attempted to cover the gamut of Dramatic Fine Spies's.

They also cover the major categories of diagnoses beloved of the "What's Wrong with You?" model: thus cases depicting depression, anxiety, alcohol dependence, personality disorder, schizophrenia and drug dependence. Embedded in each case study are clinical strategies and techniques that I have found to be helpful, but the overriding therapeutic strategy is the building of a relationship that offers empathy, curiosity, acceptance, playfulness and love. Which is, of course, PLACE - the very things that people with mental health disorders got much too little of.

Chapter Four

The teacher

It's always good to start at the beginning.

It's Glasgow, a Saturday morning in late November 1974. I'm standing outside the Glasgow University chapel. It's freezing cold. The grey black sky is spitting ice. I have in my hand a certificate (in Latin) saying I have a Master's degree in Psychological Medicine. It's official. I'm a Clinical Psychologist. The certificate is impressive. I still have it.

On that bleak day, I not only had that seemingly all-important certificate in my hand, but as of the coming Monday, I had a job to go to, as a Clinical Psychologist (albeit probationer level) in a teaching hospital. I was twenty-five years old.

I'm to be based in the Psychology Department at The Lansdowne Clinic in Glasgow with special responsibilities for the management of alcoholism. In accord with the thinking of the day, there was a brand new Alcoholism Treatment Unit in the adjacent psychiatric asylum, impressively titled Gartnavel Royal Hospital. New staff had been recruited. Me being one of them. Except … I knew nothing, nothing, nothing at all, about alcoholism.

I had rent to pay.

Alcoholism had not been mentioned on my course at all. I had done lots of study on anxiety, depression, phobias, schizophrenia, neuropsychology, even a little on psychopathy, plus lots of psychological testing, but, nothing, nothing at all, about drugs or alcohol. I knew nothing.

My childhood hadn't helped either. I have images of my father and mother arguing. My father was a very senior police officer. On seeing a drunk man he'd say, "Oh, I'll radio in and get someone to arrest him."

My mother, a social worker, saying, "No, no, he's sick, he needs to go to hospital." Meanwhile, aged about 14 and sitting silently in the back of the car, I was thinking, "You're both wrong."

Well, perhaps I knew a little.

Believe me, being a brand new, baby psychologist, was (and I'm sure for most newly qualified psychologists or counsellors of any ilk, still is), a very challenging gig. You have to try and impart to patients and staff (especially) that you know what you are doing. But you really don't. I didn't have a clue.

Looking back from the vantage point of forty-nine years in therapy, on that November day, I actually had no idea whatsoever.

However, over the following decades, I was going to learn lots. Mostly from the clients I saw. This book, to borrow a phrase, is their story.

In time, I think I got quite good at this psychotherapy game, but then again, ninety per cent of Clinical Psychologists believe they are above average therapists.

Given my initial ignorance, every new patient was daunting. "Will I be able to help?" "Will I understand what is going on?" "Am I an imposter?" "Can I use the tools I have been given?" "Will I get them better?" "I'm out of my depth."

I'm also English, so working in the west end of Glasgow I had an extra handicap - Glaswegian, "What the fuck were they saying?"

However, shifting focus away from my ineptitude, the mid 1970s, in mental health at least, was an extremely interesting time. Psychiatry was, at the time, being beguiled by psychopharmacology. In the previous twenty years there had been a revolution of new drugs. "Anti-psychotics" (Chlorpromazine, 1952) "anti-depressants" (Nardil, 1957, Imipramine, 1958) and anti-anxiety drugs (Chlordiazepoxide, 1955) had been introduced. Psychiatrists were abandoning being talking therapists and stampeding to biological explanations and solutions for mental health disorders. A biological cul-de-sac, from which few, if any, have subsequently escaped.

Yet their exodus left a vacuum for people like me and my psychology mates. We had our own holy grail. Initially, it was Behaviour Therapy and then, the real bees-knees, Cognitive Behaviour Therapy (CBT). My recently graduated colleagues and I delighted in the certainty of our new found ways. Out with psychoanalytical psychotherapy (a Prof. Eysenck had told us it didn't work and we believed him), and in with new, improved, effective CBT. Given our naivety and self-doubt, we clung to this with a desperate bravado and certainty.

Nonetheless every new referral was fraught with challenge. Would this new way be embraced by our clients? Would they delight in the magic bullets I had to offer? Could I get my patients to act their way into new ways of being?

There is now fascinating evidence about psychotherapy and what makes an effective therapist. It would have been very helpful for me if that evidence had been available in 1974.

In 2012 the American Psychological Association released a position paper on psychotherapy. They said that psychotherapy works. People who access psychotherapy do better than those who do not. About seventy percent of people engaging in psychotherapy report having benefitted from it. This is a higher good outcome rate than, for example, people visiting a cardiologist. As a talking therapist, this is very heartening news.

However, the APA also acknowledged what for them must have been, as the leading trade union for practising psychologists, a very uncomfortable truth: that your level of training, professional discipline, psychotherapeutic orientation, age, gender, and years of experience were not in any way related to the good outcomes achieved.

Well, there's a problem. All the things that psychologists hold dear and puff their chests out about, do not, when it comes to delivering effective talking therapy, seem to matter.

So, I questioned somewhat vexedly, if nine years of university education, plus lots of additional training and professional development are irrelevant, then what makes a person a good talking therapist? What makes someone an excellent psychotherapist?

I now know the answer to this because I've had the delight of listening to Dr. Scott Miller talk about his research into the making of supershrinks.

Actually, it's a good, funny story. Well, the way he tells it, it is.

It goes like this. Scott Miller was interested in the fact that when you compare two active brands of psychotherapy against each other, the outcomes, even from quite diverse interventions, come out about the same. For example, in Project Match, one of the largest psychotherapy studies ever undertaken, one thousand alcohol dependent patients were randomly allocated to four interventions. These interventions varied from CBT, to the theoretically very different Twelve-Step therapy.

On follow-up, the results from the four different approaches were the same. About seventy percent of the patients did well.

Intriguingly though, when the therapist's outcomes were considered, it was very evident that some therapists, irrespective of type of therapy, did better than some of their same brand peers. Thus, there were effective CBT therapists and effective Twelve-Step therapists and also, irrespective of brand of therapy, poor therapists. Each type of therapy seemed to have its stars and dullards.

This result was exactly the same as in the famous, and much argued over, NIMH study into depression. In this 1985 treatment study, CBT was pitted against interpersonal psychotherapy and two forms of generic clinical management that included the prescription of an "anti-depressant." All did equally well.

This equivalence in outcome, which is a consistent finding when two or more active therapies undertaken by practitioners skilled in their particular form of therapy are compared, has been summarised by noting that "all have done well and all deserve prizes."

Nonetheless, still within such comparisons some therapists are more effective than their peers.

So Dr. Scott Miller and his colleagues from the Institute for the Study of Therapeutic Change in Chicago decided it was time to determine what made some people better therapists than others. So they visited lots of different counselling agencies and videotaped hundreds of counselling sessions. They then viewed the resulting videos to see what the secret, magic ingredient was.

It was, well, not obvious. Despite lots of time, money, effort and thinking, the elusive "what makes one therapist better than another" remained unanswered.

Scott Miller then told this story, which is so good that it could possibly be true.

Scott Miller reported that he was flying back to Chicago from a meeting in Norway and was agonising about what it was in those videos he and his team had missed. Why were they no closer to the answer about what makes a therapist a good one? Were all the hours of work, never mind the research money, going to count for naught?

Somewhat despondent, he started to talk to the passenger next to him. It eventually transpired that his fellow passenger was an author, who just happened to be working on a book about excellence. Scott Miller reported that he was on to this in a flash.

"What sort of excellence?" he keenly asked.

"Oh, excellence across the board, excellence in general," was the reply.

"Have you looked at psychotherapy?"

"No," replied the fellow traveller, "but psychotherapists would no doubt be the same as every other form of excellence, they're human too."

Scott Miller said he held his breath and quietly asked. "Are you saying that excellent surgeons, ballerinas, cardiologists, singers, psychologists, football players and painters all excel for the exact same reason?"

"Yes, of course," came the reply, "excellence is achieved by the same method whatever the field."

Desperately, Miller asked, "And what is that?"

The answer to his prayers, his worries, his research grant, his career, was a sentence away.

"Ah," said his fellow traveller, "you'll have to buy the book, it's called *The Cambridge Book of Excellence,* it's coming out soon." Then promptly fell asleep.

In fact, as Scott Miller later found, what makes people excellent is practice. But, not just practice. What makes people excellent is practice with feedback; feedback from very knowledgeable sources.

WHAT HAPPENED?

I heard Scott Miller say this in a conference in California. For those of you interested in psychotherapy, the Evolution of Psychotherapy conference that is held in Annaheim every four years is very well worth a visit. In classic American, narcissistic style, it's titled an International conference, yet it only has North American speakers (a bit like the World Series). Quibbling apart, it is four days of excellence.

Interestingly, while flying home from the conference, I watched a documentary on the Australian concert pianist David Helfgott. David's life was portrayed in the Oscar winning film *Shine,* but what was of interest in this documentary was that cameras followed David Helfgott through a European recital tour. In accord with *The Cambridge Book of Excellence,* at every rehearsal before another gig, David had someone, a conductor or a fellow musician, critique his playing. He really is quite excellent.

In Clinical Psychology much use is made of supervisors. Taking your cases to an experienced supervisor is a key part of training. However, what Scott Miller has shown is that the best feedback you get on your practice is not from a supervisor, but from your patients. The best therapists actively pursue and cultivate their clients' feedback on their work.

Scott Miller has produced a four dimension session rating form, that at the end of each session you can invite your client to fill in and rate the session they have just had. If, on any dimension, you fall below a nine out of ten rating, then you enquire of the patient, what did you need to do to improve? What would, for example, have made that rating of six a ten?

The four dimensions are:

I did not feel heard, understood and respected	I felt heard, understood and respected
We did not work on or talk about what I wanted to work on	We did work on or talk about what I wanted to work on
The therapist's approach is not a good fit for me	The therapist's approach is a good fit for me
There was something missing in the session today	Overall today's session was right for me

Justine was a Clinical Psychologist who asked me for supervision. Her biggest concern was that she knew she was censorious at times, and had a tendency to lay down the law with clients. Her father, a military man, had very strict ideas about how things needed to be done. She was also concerned that she seemed to rub some clients the wrong way and they did not return.

"What," she asked, "am I doing wrong?"

Enlightened by Scott Miller, I said, "Don't ask me ask them!"

So, at the end of each of her next one hundred sessions she did. She invited her clients to complete the Scott Miller session rating scale. One thing stood out. She always got good scores on three, but in her desire to be perfect (critical fathers have a lot to answer for), she often drove her own agenda too hard and did not focus enough on what the client wanted. So her scores on the second dimension were often low.

In the end the solution was simple. With practice and expert consumer feedback she has become a much sought-after therapist. Her return rate is literally one hundred per cent. I wonder if that is all the training neophyte therapists need, practice and feedback from clients?

In a similar vein I was once at a conference and an experienced and excellent therapist was asked what she thought was "the most important factor in making a therapist a very good one?"

Without hesitation she said, "Having a narcissistically depressed mother."

Think about it, practice with constant critical feedback!

But, of course, back in 1974, none of us knew about such things. It would have made my life much simpler if I had.

My clinical duties at the time normally involved being a co-therapist, in the mornings, doing group psychotherapy in the inpatient Alcoholism Treatment Unit. Usually, my co-therapist was, thank god, a much more experienced (by nine months) trainee psychiatrist, so it was really the blind leading the drunk - but we both learned lots.

In the afternoons, I had individual clients in The Lansdowne Clinic, a beautiful old Victorian building a short walk from the main hospital. I can remember walking down from the hospital with some sense of anxiety about how the afternoon's, individual, work might go. For a start would the patient turn up? (Patient retention is a key marker of therapist effectiveness). Would there be any nasty (beyond my competence) surprises?

Then this happened, another very important lesson delivered and slowly learned.

The afternoon in question was relatively benign. I had a psychometric assessment to conduct and then one individual session. The psychometric assessment was easy. As students we had been over-trained on the Wechsler Adult Intelligence Scale, the Rey Visual Picture and the Wechsler Memory Scale. In those days, before CAT scans and MRIs were invented, Clinical Psychologists were the go-to people for any questions concerning cognitive competence. I liked the notion that I could determine, for any given patient, whether there was an organic (brain) problem or a functional (mental health) issue. It's good to be able to contribute, especially when you're not really sure you do. However, most of the results indicated a psychological issue of unknown aetiology.

My 4pm patient was Mary, a twenty-eight-year-old primary school teacher. Mary had been referred for CBT to manage her depression that had insidiously developed following the death of her mother some four years earlier. I had been seeing her regularly for about six months. We had worked well together.

Mary came in and sat down. I welcomed her with my standard opening.

"How's your world?" I said to Mary.

It's very useful to have a standard opening question. First, patients get used to it, know what to expect and can, if they wish, come to session with an answer that sets the agenda for the session. Secondly, if you ask the same question of the same patient over several sessions you get to know how they usually respond, so deviance from the normal is a useful signal. Similarly, if you ask the same question enough times of different patients then any odd answers stand out and can guide you to important therapeutic issues.

As it happens I have two standard opening questions, one for new patients and one for regular patients.

My opening question for a new patient is:

"Welcome, now what brings you to see a psychologist?"

This usually prompts the patient to identify a significant issue and offers a good place to start.

I only once had the reply: "I came by bus."

He wasn't being funny and that instantly told me lots about that client.

The very eminent American psychotherapist, Dr. Irvin Yalom, apparently asks, "What ails you?"

I have tried this twice.

The first time the patient was bewildered "Ails? Ails? What are you talking about?" Not a good start.

The second said: "Oh, I don't drink, doc!" No better.

Nevertheless, the point of both these opening questions is that right from the outset the client is invited to portray their world as they see it. Thus, we go where they want to go.

Mary was a repeat patient so I asked, "How's your world?"

Mary looked at me and smiled. She said, "Good!"

"Oh, we can't have that!" I joked, playfully.

"I have exciting news," said Mary.

"Pray tell."

"I have just been offered a job in London and I've accepted it!"

"Ha, well done. When are you thinking of leaving?"

"Next week," she laughed. "So, this is our last session."

We spent the rest of the session exploring the ramifications of her move. Was her on and off again partner going to London?

"No." (Excellent, I thought. I was convinced that he contributed to Mary's low opinion of herself).

"What was her biggest concern about going to London?"

"Leaving dad." (Ah, another draining obligation).

"What was she looking forward to?"

"Being unknown and being able to be anyone I want." (Great, freedom at last!)

What had become apparent in our sessions was that Mary, an only child, had been brought up in an emotionally volatile household. Although a caring father, Mary described her dad as being at times "bitter, mean-spirited, truculent and dangerous." Her mother was a demure, eager to please woman, who cowed in front of her husband's occasional outbursts of rancour. Mary had taken on the role from a very early age of being the go-between, the United Nations, domestic peace-keeper. She became skilled at pacifying, of protecting her mother and putting her parents' needs ahead of her own. She was very adept at deferring, demurring, de-escalating and accepting the obligations of her existence. Going to London was a truly radical step.

This final session sped by. Just before the end I asked, "Mary, can you fill in this depression scale for me? It's the same one that you filled in when we started."

Test, then post-test; we had after all been trained in the "scientist-practitioner" model.

Her scores reflected her presentation. On intake she was on the border between moderately and severely depressed. Today, she was at the low end of a bit depressed.

I said to her, "Mary, you've done really well. Can I ask you a few questions about the work we did in our sessions together? It would help me know what worked for you."

She acquiesced.

"Now, Mary, if you think about the work we did how important was the Mood Diary?"

"Ah," said Mary, "look, I never really kept that, I just wrote it up the night before coming to see you."

We had in our training been warned about patients not doing their homework, but I had forgotten to check.

"Okay, how about the activity scheduling work?"

"Ah, sorry Bill, I filled that in along with the diary!"

(Note to self: I really must be more vigilant about patient compliance).

"And the pleasure and mastery scales?"

Mary looked down. "Same," she said. "I just fudged them."

"Ha" I said, quietly confident, "Then, it was the automatic negative thought recognition strategies that we used?"

Mary had been a great one for saying "I think he thinks this or I think she thinks that" and such thoughts were always to Mary's detriment. We had worked very hard on that. I'd had fun telling her that what other people think doesn't matter. Mind you, I hadn't been brought up by Mary's father.

Mary paused. "Well, not really Bill, that's just the way I think."

I was, at this point, bewildered.

"So, Mary," I somewhat tetchily asked, "Why do you think you got better?"

"That's easy," said Mary, "I thought you liked me."

I looked at her, amazed. "Yes," I said, "I do."

And I did.

Ha, there was some really excellent feedback.

Psychotherapy works because a positive attachment is formed. Therapy works because the client can experience a place of acceptance, of being safe, of being heard, of being interesting, important, attuned to and valued. Some or all of which were missing in their childhoods. Psychotherapy is restorative; good therapy gives clients what they didn't get: in Mary's case, that was not enough of the right stuff.

Chapter Five

Once were reptiles

In the understanding of the impact of trauma on adult emotional regulation, it is useful to have an understanding of how our emotions work. The extent and degree of your childhood adversity is critical. The worse your childhood the more likely you will be to undone by your emotions. Bessel van der Kolk asserts that you are more likely to have long term problems with the regulation of emotions such as sexual impulses, anxiety and anger, if trauma occurred at a young age. The younger the age, and the longer the duration of the trauma, then the likelihood of issues with emotional regulation increases, especially emotions like anger and anxiety.

Anger is very interesting; it is the marker emotion, the emotion that shows your childhood up. The best test of how well you emotionally regulate yourself is how well do you manage your anger?

If you've ever screamed "fuck you!" at a partner, friend, child, sibling, colleague, fellow road user, or indeed anyone at all, then your childhood was not optimum. You have trouble with emotional regulation.

If you've never done that, well, well done. Very well done. You were lucky, you had a good childhood. Thank mum and dad now.

Screaming "fuck you" at someone, often feels in the moment totally right. They had it coming, they absolutely deserved it.

However, did that expletive bullet really work? Did it get you what you wanted from your outburst? Or, somehow did your righteous indignation and rageful venom obscure the legitimacy of your case?

Did that well merited "fuck you" perversely *fuck you*?

There is an art to anger; an art to making it work for you. There is also a dark side to anger that can literally destroy your life, so it is important to understand anger. In order to do so it is necessary to reflect on our emotions.

WHAT HAPPENED?

There are seven universal emotions. That is emotions we all have. Anger is one of them. Anger is in all of us, along with the other six. Have a go at naming them.

They are love, anxiety, shame, sadness, joy, and surprisingly, surprise.

If you look at this list of ill-sorted emotional bedfellows, what strikes you about them?

Most clients on seeing this list go "what about …?" and name other emotions.

For example, when running a group for depressed patients there will always be a clamour to include guilt. No, it's not on the universal list, not everyone does guilt. Or, the "lessnesses" - a powerful cadre of personal melancholia, yet there are no uselessnesses, powerlessnesses, hopelessnesses or worthlessnesses, on the universal list.

One patient bitterly commented, "All the emotions I have trouble with aren't on that list." Another impatiently quipped, "I don't want any of them! Can I give them back?" Or, "What use are they?" "Why do we have them?"

Good question, why do we have them? The answer is strangely simple. The universal emotions are essential for our survival.

Love ensures the evolution of our species, anxiety warns us of danger, joy tells us we are doing something right, sadness helps us manage loss, surprise orientates us, and anger can energise us into protective action.

So rather than anger being a bad, unhelpful or an unnecessary emotion, anger is right up there with the best of them, such as love or joy. Like the other six universal emotions, anger is a vital part of our human make-up. We literally cannot live without it. Anger protects us, gives us enormous drive to defend ourselves, propels us to fight off attacks and prompts us to right wrong-doing.

So don't leave home without it.

Clearly, anger is not always useful. Indeed, anger that tips into violence is not usually species enabling. But if you are Scottish and the Vikings are marauding up the beach, a bit of angry violence may come in handy.

However, the anger that generates domestic violence, one-hit punches, prolonged assaults or traumatises children, is anger at its worst.

The key is that for emotions to be survival-enhancing, literally to be good, useful emotions, they have to felt *cleanly*. They have to be instantly recognised by the person, and in this recognition, direction and energy can be achieved. Thus, universal emotions felt cleanly are organising. They literally tell us what to do.

Anger is exactly the same as the other the essential seven. It can be organising or disorganising. Anger that is felt cleanly is helpful. But usually that "fuck you" anger is disorganised anger.

Think about the last time you literally lost it. How quickly did your anger/rage come on?

Were you calm one moment, yelling the next?
Were you taken by surprise by your own anger?
Did you feel irritated and out of sorts afterwards?
Did your rage invalidate any legitimacy in your shift to anger?

Answer yes to any of the above and your anger is not clean anger. It is disorganised anger, messy, unhelpful anger. It's anger that you need to do something about, because *it will damage your life.*

Let's take Davis as an example. He was referred to me by his GP and the letter stated that although Davis was a successful academic (he was a Professor of Psychology!), he needed help managing his anger.

When I asked him the standard "what brings you to see a psychologist" question, his reply was "You know I am a psychologist don't you?"

Such non sequitur replies are delightful, because they are indicators that something is amiss. There is an issue that needs to be addressed. I could feel his embarrassment at being a psychologist and needing to see a psychologist, and perhaps underneath his embarrassment at coming to seeing a psychologist at all.

I said, "Yes, and how awkward are you feeling about being a psychologist and coming to see one?"

"Very," he said. "I think I should have been able to work out for myself why at times I get so angry. I've had a complaint at work and my wife and kids don't like it," and, he paused, "and it's not befitting someone of my status."

I felt for him and his enormously erroneous idea that "people of status" are all emotionally regulated creatures.

But one thing at a time, so I said, "Tell me about your anger, can you give me a recent example when you got really angry?"

He told me that some two weeks previously on a Saturday morning he had dropped his two daughters off for netball and then, having some free time, had decided to go for a swim and a coffee. On his way to the pool he happened to pass a large stationery store and on impulse he had driven in. He said that he needed a few things and was very pleased that he was able to park right by the entrance and then discovered that everything he wanted was right to hand and some items were even discounted. He said that he was looking forward to his swim and then a coffee and that he felt that "the world was a good place." But then he reported it all went rapidly wrong.

He said that as he approached the checkout, the phone by the till rang. Despite two staff members happily chatting nearby, the till operator answered the phone. It quickly became clear that the till operator was a bit of a wiz on the complexities of printing over-sized documents. He happily gave a colleague helpful advice.

WHAT HAPPENED?

However, he didn't serve Davis. Davis said that although he gestured to the till operator that he wanted to buy the items he was holding the till operator merely nodded and continued talking. Davis said that he could feel himself becoming agitated. So he turned and walked toward another till that was empty. As he approached, the operator walked off. Davis said that he had politely asked, "Oh, could I buy these please?" The staff member's response was that she was going on her break and that Davis should use the other open till. When Davis looked back the other till operator was still on the phone enthusiastically imparting advice.

Now an emotionally regulated shopper would quietly have approached the two still chatting employees and asked for service. But, not Davis. He said that he put his potential purchases on the ground, jumped onto an adjacent (low) table and at the top of his lungs had enquired to everyone, "How the fuck does anyone get service in this fucking shop?"

He reported that he had duly pointed out that the staff seemed to be more interested in chatting, going on breaks or advising a colleague, than actually selling anything. He had pointed out that if it wasn't for the likes of him, they wouldn't have a job, and how the fuck did they think that not taking money from anyone was good for the fucking business. Or, he said "words to that general effect."

Apparently when Davis had stopped ranting there had been a stunned awkward silence. The till/phone man then quietly put down his phone and beckoned Davis over. In total silence the sale of Davis' purchases was completed.

However, just as Davis was walking away, the till operator had said to him, "You have a better day now!"

Davis said that despite the rightness of his position (after all, selling things are what shops are about!), he had left the store feeling undone. His righteous indignation, his rabid rage, had eventually got him served, but he was also sure that the staff had banded together later over a "he was a fucking nutter" conversation.

Davis said that somehow he had, despite being right, invalidated himself. Davis said that his swim was dismal, the coffee was awful and that he had spent the afternoon ruminating on the incident.

That's the trouble with disorganised anger. It invalidates you. It really is a "fuck you" that fucks you.

Davis said that to make matters worse, when he later collected his daughters and was asked how his morning had been, he had to reluctantly acknowledge that he had had an altercation in a shop. Apparently his children had looked at each other and his oldest daughter had said, "Well, that's another store we can't go into again." They had then conspired happily together and recalled other instances of Davis' altercations in stores.

Davis then said that the final straw was when his youngest daughter had, with a glint of teenage innocent delight, said, "Hey, Dad, do you think there's a theme here?"

Which was why Davis was now sitting in front of me. Why did he keep on doing this?

Well, the answer, of course, lay in "what had happened to him."

In order to understand outbursts of anger (or rage) like Davis' it is necessary to have some understanding of how our brains work and why rage happens.

Simply put, we have three brains. We have a reptilian brain, a mammalian brain and a logical brain. They are of course connected, but none controls the others.

The oldest is our reptilian brain. We once were reptiles. Reptiles are on their own from the outset.

Turtles are reptiles. Mummy turtle comes ashore, clambers up the beach, digs a big hole and deposits a multitude of fertilised eggs. She then scarpers back to the relative safety of the deep oceans.

When they hatch, baby turtles have one primitive purpose, to survive. Thus, they get into the water as quickly as possible and do their utmost to avoid being eaten alive by the waiting pack of predators. Unfortunately, even the sea is not safe. The survival rate of baby turtles is less than two percent. No wonder their reptilian brains are working overtime. They must scamper down the beach and into the ocean with their brains going, "run, run, run, run."

We still have remnants of reptilian brain. It does exactly the same as the turtles'. It looks for threats to our existence. When it spots such, it works lightning fast to try and avoid destruction. Indeed, our reptilian brains work quicker than our later acquired thinking, logical, brain.

To illustrate the superiority of our reptilian brain, imagine the following. You are sitting on the couch at home and a tiger walks in. If you wonder "oh my goodness what's a tiger doing in suburbia?" you will get eaten.

Such thinking is not helpful, but fleeing or freezing is. Your reptilian brain will do that for you. The important point is that like it or not, when under a threat, your reptilian brain works quicker than you can think about it. The rapidity of its action may save your life.

Unfortunately, our brilliant, rapidly responding, life-saving reptilian brains can also be very problematic. Anyone who works with offenders will hear stories of inexplicable violence.

Phil is a case in point. I was asked by his lawyer to prepare a psychological report; to attempt some explanation of Phil's recent violent behaviour and his re-offending risk.

Phil was playing pool with a friend on a Friday night in his local pub. Another patron came up to the table and placed a coin on the table indicating to Phil that he wanted the next game. Five minutes later Phil, without warning, ran to the potential pool player and beat him unconscious with his pool cue.

In doing the report I explored Phil's history. He was born in Manchester and he and his brother lived in what he described as a "Coronation Street." His childhood was tough and not helped by his father's anger, difficulty in keeping a job and the occasional outbreaks of parental domestic violence.

However, Phil also reported that from the age of ten until he was fourteen, his mum used to attend night school, on a Friday night. She was studying to become a nurse. A goal she eventually achieved when Phil was fourteen. So every Friday for four years Phil would leave school, go to his grandmother's and wait for his dad to pick him up. Every Friday Phil's dad would turn up on his motorcycle and Phil would catch a pillion ride home.

Every Friday, dad would stop two streets away from home and tell Phil to run up through a pedestrian pass and get home as quickly as he could. Dad would then roar off on his bike and race him to the house. Every Friday, no matter how fast Phil ran, how hard he tried, dad always got there first. The penalty for coming second was that Phil was marched into the back garden and thrashed with a length of hose filled with sand. Phil noted that when he was being beaten, his dad always "zoned out" and "looked as though he wasn't there."

When I asked Phil to explain to me why he had assaulted the stranger. Phil said, "Well, he looked at me funny."

We both understood that on that Friday night in a pub, the stranger waiting for his game of pool, probably conveying some impatience at having to wait, just for a moment looked like dad about to deliver a thrashing.

I pondered whether Phil had a chance. His reptilian brain did what reptilian brains always do. When sensing a significant threat they act; without thinking, or more correctly, before thinking. When our reptilian brains get triggered it is a matter of "shoot first, ask questions later." Phil was sentenced to seven years imprisonment for aggravated assault.

About a million years ago we developed as mammals. Baby mammals get suckled, nurtured, and protected. We were no longer cast aside to look after ourselves. Now, nurturance was needed, nurturance was all. Nurturance is the key to survival and to emotional regulation.

Over my career I must have written over a thousand court reports. Reports requested by lawyers for the defence, the prosecution or the court itself to bring a psychological explanation to the offending. Some crimes have been major: murder, rape, aggravated assault, drug importation, arson, deprivation of liberty; some more mundane, shoplifting, drunk driving, fraud, theft, possession with intent to supply, and one a delightful, "deliberately driving too slowly" charge.

Yet in all of these reports I have never written something like, "Fred had a lovely childhood, and then at the age of eighteen he started assaulting grandmothers."

Every court report I have ever written has included a history of childhood neglect and or abuse. Every single one.

If we wish to lower the crime rate then the most effective crime prevention initiative would be to ensure that any child exhibiting unusual behaviours (acting out or acting in) at school would prompt a supportive intervention in the home and the school. Similarly, any drug harm reduction strategy needs to start with understanding that if you have had a good enough childhood then drugs will not be a problem. The answer is not more police officers, more sniffer dogs, longer sentences, bigger jails, more tough love, rather, right from the outset, we need initiatives that improve the quality of everyone's childhood.

Within our mammalian brains we all have an amygdala. Your amygdala is a bit like a smoke detector. Smoke detectors are alert all the time and constantly sense for that which they don't want to sniff; the smell and the chemicals of smoke. When they do detect smoke they set off a piercing alarm, the sound of which brings to your attention that you are in danger; hopefully, before the house burns down. Yet often there are false alarms.

Your amygdala, nestled in the inner surface of your temporal lobes, is just like a smoke detector. It sits like an island in a river of information constantly monitoring what is going on, internally and externally.

Just for a moment sit still, shut your eyes and monitor yourself. How is the saliva in your mouth? How clenched are your teeth? Feel the palms of your hands, dry or moist? How is your pulse rate? How is your breathing? What can you hear? What can you see? What can you smell? What can you taste? How do you feel? How tense are you? How is your inner world? How is the outer world? Surprising, what's going on is totally unnoticed, isn't it?

Your amygdala never sleeps. It is on guard 24/7, monitoring every aspect of your being that you just take for granted.

It is possible, using different type of brain imaging, to show that the amygdalae of young children who are neglected and/or abused respond differently to the amygdalae of nurtured children. The neglected, abused children are more reactive, because their stress fight/flight reaction has been more frequently tripped. As has been sagely noted by Donald Hebb, "neurons that fire together wire together." Thus, children from neglected and/or abusive backgrounds have different wiring and different trip patterns, both from nurtured children and each other. No two brains are wired the same. No two amygdalae are the same.

This, of course, explains why the search for the biological cause of mental illnesses keeps failing. There is not a distinctive pattern, even of childhood trauma, because everyone's experiences of trauma are different. Our brains are all individually wired.

A study comes to mind. It is known as the 9/11 study. Following the attack on the twin towers in New York researchers tracked down fifty women who had not only been present at what became later known as ground zero, as workers, shoppers, coffee drinkers or first responders, but who were at the time also pregnant. The researchers matched these women to fifty other pregnant New Yorkers, but the difference was on that day they were not in Manhattan and had not been directly involved in the destruction of the twin towers.

Five years later they interviewed and examined the children of these one hundred mothers. What became evident was that children of the women who had been directly involved in 9/11 were, in comparison to the not-involved children, more anxious, had higher autonomic arousal and reactivity and were hypervigilant. This may sound problematic, but actually these responses were adaptive. These children had been prepared for a dangerous world, whereas the children of non-involved mothers had been prepared for a safer one. It's that difference between wired for connection versus wired for protection.

So we have these individually-wired amygdalae that respond differently to the world. The trouble for traumatised people is that when their amygdala get activated it is distressing because, just like fire alarms, there is the perception of a serious threat.

Our amygdalae learn well and quickly. So, a person who has, as she slipped into unconsciousness while being raped and strangled, heard a wind chime, will later in life dissociate or flee at the sound of a wind chime.

Another patient got herself into trouble because while in hospital and watching an episode of *Special Victims' Unit* (an American crime show involving sexual crimes), she became very distressed. A child rape victim herself, her very evident distress prompted an Italian male patient to go to the kitchen and find her some cake. Now we have two childhoods at work. When the male patient insisted she have some cake ("I wanted to soothe her"), she eventually punched him, breaking his nose. "He wouldn't take no for an answer," was her answer. Such are our amygdalae.

Every now and then in couples therapy I am reminded that all marriages are but collisions of childhoods. Mario and Simone, a recently married couple, came to therapy because of their terrible fights. Each accused the other of being rageful. At one session they described a ferocious fight that had ended with Simone packing her bags and going to stay with friends, from where she had only just returned.

Mario was a second generation Italian migrant and his father had, like most of the post-war migrants from Italy, arrived in Australia with nothing. They then worked extraordinarily hard at making a place for their families. Mario's father had been a carpenter and had drilled into Mario from a very early age that your tools were to be cherished, looked after and valued, because they were the means to your survival. He had on occasions literally beaten this knowledge into his son.

Simone, also of European extraction, had been brought up in a large family where food was much treasured as a way of celebrating family life. Their last fight had happened because Simone, keen to demonstrate her love to Mario, was preparing his favourite lunch; a continental roll filled with cheese, meat and pickles. Meanwhile Mario was sitting happily chatting to his wife when to his horror and rage, Simone struggling to open a jar of pickles, picked up a knife from the very expensive set of kitchen knives given as a wedding present by Mario's father, and stabbed the lid of the pickle jar with the precious knife. Mayhem ensued.

The trouble is that because there are no actual, real rules for life, we all learn our own set of rules as children, which are always different from those of our partners.

There is another issue to add to this complexity in that we have three brains. The third is our front brain, also known as our logical brain. On a good day, under normal circumstances, the front brain rules. It is logical, it is calm. It is also our supervisor, our good brain. It helps us appreciate that our urges need not be attended to, be that an attractive cake, person, dress or car. Furthermore, the odd pang of jealously or wave of sadness coming up from our emotional brain can be reasoned with, explained and tucked away.

Yet when things go wrong and the amygdala sees a threat, it instantly provokes our reptilian brain into action. "Shoot first, ask questions later," may save your life. Unfortunately, this is the exact scenario that results in armed, but under perceived threat, police officers killing innocent people.

Now think of the last time you lost it. You know, went ape shit, had a meltdown, went from calm to rage in a nanosecond. Where did you feel it?

What is fascinating is that when the amygdala trips our reptilian brain into action, there is a felt physical reaction. Some people will report feeling it in their stomach, for others "it's a punch in the chest," and some say they feel it in their heads or their throats. Wherever it is, it is a vital visceral warning that you are about to act out (rage, anger, expletives), or act in (freeze, go mute or numb).

For the "act outers," here is your signal that in the next moment you will lash out. But, because our reptilian brains are wired to protect us it is difficult to sense that physical event and catch ourselves in time. Ah, so there you go again.

The trick is to understand what your amygdala picked up. Why did it react just then? What old wound got reactivated?

WHAT HAPPENED?

The thing is, if you can gain some understanding as to the trigger, then you may be able to use your logic brain and your emotional brain to slow down, maybe even turn off, that reptilian rush to rage.

So back to Davis and his rage, we explored his childhood, which he said was "Okay." He had a PLACE score in the mid-teens so not that crash hot, but "okay."

His mother was a legal secretary and his father a remote, often absent, civil engineer. Born in England, Davis' family had migrated to Australia when he was thirteen. He noted that the transition from the UK to Australia was difficult. Many of the things he had enjoyed in England (especially soccer) were absent in his new land. He also struggled to fit in with what he considered the too lazy, liberal, easy-going pace of his new school peers, who preferred surfing to studying. So Davis said his teens were quite solitary, but once he attended university he managed to establish and maintain a small cadre of friends, including one who became his wife.

When we explored, he did report that during this time there were occasional outbursts of anger (really rage) and usually they related to being in shops, cafeterias and pubs. Davis noted that because these outbursts were occasional, his rage had little impact on his work or domestic life. He said most of the time he was emotionally very well-mannered.

He proudly reported that he had been the top student in his final undergraduate year and had immediately done a PhD, while working as an occasional lecturer. He then noted that he had had a very successful three years lecturing at a university in the UK before coming back to Australia for his current professorial post.

When we explored his rage we would return to the same impasse. He was ninety-nine percent of the time an easy-going man of a happy disposition who got on reasonably well with most people. He reported that in his childhood nothing untoward had happened. Well, a priest had attempted to rape him when he was aged fourteen, but he had managed to escape from the situation unscathed.

The cause of his rage remained hidden. Trauma breeds rage, so what had happened to Davis?

Sometimes it is necessary to dig deep. Trauma is often repressed and pushed down well below the surface. Buried deep but not, if approached adroitly, totally hidden.

So I encouraged Davis to practice "ocean breathing." Borrowed from the Comprehensive Resource Model, ocean breathing is visualising you are standing by an ocean and breathing continuous cycles of air in through your nose and then out of your mouth.

It's very relaxing, very calming and, with practice, mildly hypnotic.

Davis enjoyed ocean breathing and was able to get into relaxed space quickly.

Then in one session, I said to him, "Keep your eyes closed, now tell me what colour you see in front of your eyes."

"Red," he said.

I then instructed him, "Okay, now I want you to look into that red and search for any lighter, whiter area."

I tell him to keep breathing and look for that lighter, whiter space in front of his eyes. Look for the lighter, whiter space.

"How you going in there?" I queried.

"Good," he said.

"Now," I said, "I want you, without any hesitation or restriction, to do exactly what I am going to ask."

He nodded.

"I want you to think of a number."

It's instant, "Ten," he said.

I tell him to keep breathing and then, "Again, without any hesitation or restriction, I want you to think of being ten years old," Davis nodded and I instructed him to "think of an image."

I watched Davis closely. I saw his eyes flicker and his body tense. I told him to stay with the image, and then, "What story does it tell?"

Davis sat absolutely still. A tear rolled down his cheek.

I said, "If that tear had a voice what would it say?"

Davis slowly told me. The image he had recalled was curiously an image of the car his father had when he was ten. It was a black Daimler 250 Mark II saloon.

He then told the story that throughout his childhood he had been afraid of his austere father and spent very little time with him. However, Davis said that once every fortnight he and his dad would drive to Coventry City's Football ground. On arrival there his dad would park the car, give Davis the keys and tell him to be back at the car at the end of the game. Davis said he would then join his friends at one end of the ground, while his dad would sit in the stand.

At the end of the game Davis would return quickly to the car, let himself in and wait for his father's return. Usually, this only meant waiting ten or fifteen minutes. However, Davis recalled one Saturday his father had taken over an hour to return to the car. Davis remembered being very bored and gradually more and more distressed. On his father's eventual return, Davis remembered saying something like, "Dad if you knew you were going so long you could have told me. I could have caught a bus home."

Davis said he had just remembered his father's reply. It was, "If you don't like it, don't come."

Davis said that his father's response was crushing. This was the only time he ever spent alone with his father and the message was: you don't matter. You're not important."

Davis noted that he never went to football with his father again. When twenty years later his father died, they were, to all intents and purposes, strangers.

We all have hurt buttons. Wounds from the past that when pressed can ignite us into rage. Davis' hurt button was sensing any signs that he did not matter.

Old wounds may die hard, but they can die.

That's the trick of hurt buttons. You can't manage them with logic. You have to manage them with insight, compassion and acceptance. You have to allow your emotional self to be a place of compassion and understanding that prevents old wounds tripping you into rage. So when your emotional fire alarm goes off and that physical reaction to a subliminal threat happens, you can smile to yourself and say "it's that old hurt button working." You can look around and see what the amygdala has seen, perhaps even feel the distress in your body, and then walk away. For people who have had traumatic childhoods, or as in Davis' case, a low grade childhood with a significant, accumulative, damaging event, then becoming rageful is a normal part of adult life.

After all, we once were reptiles.

Chapter Six

Getting out of jail

I was asked to see Gordon, who was, as the referring psychiatrist said, "one of your lot." By that, he meant an academic. At the time I was teaching Clinical Psychology four days a week and one day a week I was a clinician. I was sensitive to the perhaps not inaccurate taunt of "if you can, you do, if you can't, you teach."

Gordon was a professor at a different local university. A week earlier he had tried to kill himself by strapping weights to his legs and jumping into his swimming pool. This was not, as Gordon quickly discovered, a very efficient method of suicide. Every time he sank to the bottom of his pool and ran out of breath his reptilian brain activated and he automatically kicked himself upwards, gasped in air, then sank back under.

This process not only took time but became sufficiently noisy to attract the attention of a neighbour, who called an ambulance and, much to Gordon's chagrin, climbed over the fence and hauled him out.

Having introduced myself, I sat with him in his hospital room. His demeanour screamed defeat. He said that it was all too hard, he couldn't go on. He was a fake, a fraud, a failure. He said that however hard he tried he was always running on empty; he never got ahead, he was exhausted. He felt dead inside. So, he said, "I might as well be dead."

I listened to him and invited him to use his inpatient stay as a time to hibernate and literally do nothing. However, the idea was abhorrent to him.

"What of my job? I've got work to do. You don't understand, I have to keep going, I can't stop, I'll be found out!"

Ah, therein is the problem.

Depression is not a biological disorder. It is a psychological one. A British psychologist, Dorothy Rowe, has summed up depression beautifully. She wrote:

WHAT HAPPENED?

"Depression is a prison in which you are both the suffering prisoner and the cruel jailer."

Why be a cruel jailer to yourself? Well, because something happened in your childhood that *makes you* cruel to yourself. I suspected that in his protest Gordon had revealed the cause of his inhumanity to himself. Could it be that he only mattered because of what he achieved? Did his value lay in his external achievements and the good opinions of others?

As I wrote a brief record of my first contact with Gordon into his inpatient case notes I happened to see his medication sheet. I was stunned. Here was a forty-eight-year-old, high-functioning (well, up until very recently) male, who according to his drug chart, was on 80mg of Lexapro daily, 30mg of Avanza at night and 200mg of slow release Seroquel.

He was not being medicated, he was being drugged.

For those of you who are not familiar with these medications, the normal therapeutic dose range for Lexapro (an "anti-depressant") is 10mg to 20mgs per day. And although both the Avanza (a different type of "anti-depressant") and the Seroquel (an "anti-psychotic") doses were unremarkable in isolation, when taken altogether this was an unusual and problematic level of sedation.

Here is a tricky issue. As a Clinical Psychologist one is expected to leave the medication to the prescribing doctor and get on with being the therapist. This is a division of labour I like. I never have to get involved with patients haggling for more or different drugs. Furthermore, I hate it when the prescriber wants to meddle in what therapy I'm up to, or worse, have a go at some talking therapy themselves. So, there is a happy demarcation of duties - until you see that, for whatever reason, a patient is being prescribed levels of psychotropics that cannot be helpful.

And how would I know what is, or is not, helpful medication? The answer is that I made it my business to know. There is within Clinical Psychology a reluctance to be involved or become knowledgeable about psychopharmacology. Yet I think we fail to offer our patients optimum care if we do not have at least a working knowledge of what they are being prescribed and what the current issues may be.

Take the following little example. I had a fifty-five-year-old senior education administrator in group. He was an occasional attender at a men's group that ran every Monday night. When invited to reflect on how he was traveling he told the group, "It is official, I'm crazy."

He then told the following story. On awakening on the previous Sunday morning he had gone to get himself a cup of tea when he discovered much to his annoyance that the kitchen was littered with empty Indian food containers and general mess. He was even more annoyed that on independently questioning his two adult children they both vehemently denied that they had had a late night Indian food binge.

He told the group that he was sure it was his daughter who had, he said, a bit of a history of bingeing on food and then being deceptive about her behaviour. So he hit on a plan. As soon as the local Indian restaurant opened, he went and asked the proprietor, "Which one of my two children came in late last night and ordered lots of take away?"

The reply took him by total surprise. "Oh no sir, not your children sir, it was you, sir. And sir, may I request that next time you come and visit us you wear more than just your underpants?"

The group delighted in the tale and even the patient concerned smiled ruefully at the vision of himself in his underpants, at midnight, ordering three Indian meals with accompaniments.

He then talked about how distressed he was that he could do something like that and have absolutely no recall. He said he wondered whether he had a brain tumour or was totally crazy. He was visibly distressed.

I was suspicious. His presentation in the few times I had seen him was articulate, measured and insightful. His issues revolved around his relationship with his wife and their recent separation. So I asked him, "Tell me, what you do remember from that night?"

He reported that he had earlier that evening dropped his daughter off at the local train station, returned home, had dinner, a couple of glasses of wine and then watched a wildlife documentary on the Discovery channel. He said that he had gone to bed about 10pm, but because of ruminating about his relationship he couldn't get to sleep, so he had taken a sleeping pill and then fallen asleep, for what he had thought was the entire night.

"Stilnox?" I asked.

"Eh, yes," he said. "My GP prescribed it last week, first time I've used it. How did you know it was Stilnox?"

I then told him and the group Stilnox horror stories: the woman who unknowingly spray-painted her dog red, the man who missed his flight, the woman who, on a massive GP inspired dose, was so terrified to detox that she killed herself. Stilnox (aka Ambien) really is a shocker, tales like his abound.

He was not going crazy, he was just another Stilnox casualty.

Stilnox comes with a big black box warning as to its dangerousness in the prescriber's guide, the Monthly Index of Medical Specialities (MIMS), yet it is still being prescribed. My clinical experience is that it often causes dissociation and amnesia, and regular use causes benzodiazepine like dependence; a "psych med" definitely to avoid.

WHAT HAPPENED?

So in my view, it behoves all people working with clients who are taking "psych meds," to have at least a working knowledge of their impact.

This is especially so with the so-called "anti-depressants." The nomenclature used here is fascinating. We are all used to antibiotics. You get an infection, be it from bad luck or bad behaviour, and after a consultation with a doctor and maybe some pathology, an antibiotic will be prescribed that will literally kill the bug you had. Antibiotics kill bacteria and you get better. The bug is gone.

Not so with "anti-depressants." They do not kill depression they at best palliate it, or reduce the pain, but do not remove it. A bit like taking opiates for cancer pain; you get pain relief, but you die anyway.

The claim from the pharmaceutical companies is that because of your chemical imbalance, you need to take them forever. The analogy is like insulin for diabetes, but diabetes has a known biological cause. Depression does not have one. There is absolutely no evidence whatsoever that people with depression have, as is popularly believed, lower serotonin levels than anyone else. The chemical imbalance theory that is loved by pharmaceutical companies and promulgated by them to doctors and the public is completely without scientific foundation. Or, as Bonnie Burstow has so aptly written: "People being treated for mental illnesses in point of fact have normal brain chemistry, so it stands to reason that these substances themselves cause imbalances."

It is useful to firmly put to bed any notion of chemical imbalance in the cause of depression. This is a view that is so publically accepted (great marketing from Big Pharma), that when you challenge it and say it just is not so, people often get upset with you and say, "But it's a fact." Actually - it isn't!

Just recently, one woman literally said, "But I have low serotonin levels. My doctor did a blood test and told me." Um, there are no biological markers whatsoever for any of the 265 mental illnesses, including depression. There is no blood test for low serotonin levels. The doctor fibbed.

Dr David Healy, a British psychiatrist has written that the chemical imbalance theory is "bio babble."

James Davies, in his highly readable and heretical book *Cracked*, quoted the following:

"'Despite pseudoscientific terms like 'chemical imbalance' nobody really knows what causes mental illness. There's no blood test or brain scan for major depression.' (Dr. Darshak Sanghavi, Harvard Medical School)

'Chemical imbalance is sort of last century thinking.' Dr. Joseph Coyle, Professor of Neuroscience at Harvard University.

'Many neuroscientists no longer consider a chemical imbalance theory of depression and anxiety to be valid.' (Dr. David Burns, Professor of Psychiatry at Stanford University.)

'The results of decades of neurotransmitter-depletion studies point to one inescapable conclusion, low levels of serotonin, norepinephrine or dopamine do not cause depression'. Professor Kirsch, Harvard Medical School."

All of which makes the Australian Black Dog Institute's current website very interesting. If you check, it reads:

"It is likely that with most instances of clinical depression, neurotransmitter function is disrupted".

Some ideas are just too popular, or maybe just too well-promulgated.

However, the most fascinating issue about "anti-depressants" is that they are not "anti-depressants" at all. They are "serenics;" they make you serene. That is, of course, why they are the most widely prescribed drug for people with "anxiety disorders."

There are also a myriad of problems with these so-called "anti-depressants." First, the only guaranteed thing about taking an "anti-depressant" is that you will experience side effects.

These can vary from mild to severe, and include; being sedated, being aroused, having a dry mouth, fainting, problems urinating, sweating, jerking, twitching, tooth grinding, headache, migraine, blurred vision, weight gain, nausea, dissociation, depersonalisation, derealisation, nightmares, amnesia, auditory hallucinations, confusion, loss of libido, emotional blunting, restlessness-agitation-turmoil (known as akathisia), neuropathy and a doubling of the individual's suicide risk.

There is a well-recognised serotonin syndrome caused by gradual overdosing of the client. This causes a cluster of acute side effects that include shivering, sweating, confusion, tremors, restlessness and possibly death.

Then, of course, having been on them for any length of time, there are difficulties coming off. Although declared non-addictive by the drug companies, my experience with patients coming off "anti-depressants" shows that while they may not exhibit high levels of psychological reliance they certainly have physical withdrawal effects. Most commonly these include brain zaps, dizziness, panic attacks, dread, flu like symptoms, sweating, nausea, agitation, sadness and distress.

The temptation is, of course to see this as a return of the depression, but withdrawal symptoms are always the opposite to the effect of the drug. So withdrawal off a "serenic" drug causes a loss of serenity. Thus anxiety, agitation, emotional distress, nausea, nightmares, and dizziness, are the norm.

As David Healy has written, "The first point to make is that withdrawal syndromes from anti-depressants are real and in many instances more severe than many concede."

He then cited a study of healthy, non-depressed, volunteers taking Prozac and after only two weeks of use, two-thirds of them reported withdrawal on cessation.

It is important to do any such tapering with the prescribing doctor in the loop, (rather than just plot between you and the patient), as there have been reports of patients withdrawing from drugs like Lexapro being susceptible to cardiac events.

My clinical experience is that the worst thing about being on a "serenic" drug for any length of time (six months plus), is the gradual occurrence of emotional blunting, or as one patient actually accurately put it, "I now live in the land of blur."

When I first saw Gordon I wondered how much of his depression, his struggle, was serenic-induced "land of blur."

However, with Gordon, my dilemma over his medications was easily resolved. First, the admitting psychiatrist, who was new to Gordon, was also not impressed, though for a different reason. When I raised the issue of Gordon's medication with him, he agreed and said "Actually, I don't think he's really depressed, I think he's got a dependent personality disorder, so we do not need to encourage any dependency. So yes, I'll take him off."

Fortuitously, as a four-day-a-week academic and one-day-a-week clinician, Gordon lived on my way home from the university where I taught. I took the unusual step of arranging to see him twice a week at his house. In the event, this proved to be invaluable.

First, I discovered that Gordon's life was, shall I say, complicated. Although married, his wife still lived in Sydney, from where Gordon had transferred to take up his current appointment. Gordon had subsequently developed a new relationship with a member of the university's administration staff.

This was ostensibly a secret, and a secret that caused Gordon no little angst. He was very concerned that his local "friend" would leave him, and then where would he be? Or, that his wife would find out and leave him, then where would he be?

Of course this relationship was further complicated by the fact that men on serenics have a ninety percent rate of sexual dysfunction that furthered Gordon's belief that he was inadequate. This is a serious, nasty, and possibly irreversible, side effect of taking any serenics, but especially Effexor or Pristiq. Many women on these drugs report a loss of libido, difficulty in achieving orgasm or a total loss of orgasmic capacity.

However, as an aside, if you experience premature ejaculation, taking 37.5 mgs of Effexor (known in the trade as "side-effects-or") works a treat. Just don't take it for too long.

On my first visit to Gordon after his discharge, I was let into the house by

Amanda, Gordon's new girlfriend. She was greatly concerned that since his arrival home he had done very little. "He just sits and mopes and ruminates," she said.

I explored this with Gordon and with only a little bit of encouragement Gordon did the classic catastrophizing that some people are masters at. I asked him, "What was his greatest concern?"

"Losing my job," came the reply.

"Because?"

"Because, then I will not be able to pay my bills, I will become homeless, Amanda will leave me, my wife will leave me, I will be all alone and homeless. I will have to kill myself."

Phew, one step to the abyss.

If I was, as in my psychological youth, a good cognitive behaviourist, I would have got into some reassuring logic about identifying the cognitive distortions involved in this catastrophic disaster thinking and working with Gordon on correcting them.

There was a key distortion in that he was a tenured academic, so unless found guilty of a major breach of misconduct (plagiarism or a serious criminal offence), he literally had a job for life. However, I didn't go there, I went to what I thought was the heart of the matter.

Depression is, after all, a prison in which you are both the suffering prisoner and the cruel jailer.

"Gordon, tell me how long have you felt not enough?"

"From the moment I was born."

"Tell me about it."

He slowly told of his childhood. The first of two sons, his father was a very ambitious and determined cardiologist, who was academically outstanding and a brilliant surgeon. His mother was his father's practice secretary and "servant."

He recounted that all his early memories were of his mother being harassed by her dual responsibilities to his father and to her sons.

"In that order," Gordon said, "I was a burden."

Unfortunately, Gordon's younger (by eighteen months) brother had his father's driven personality and intelligence. By the time Gordon was ten his brother was doing Gordon's homework for him and was, from Gordon's perspective, the more favoured child.

I have an exercise that encapsulates the dictum that the strategies you use to stay safe psychologically as a child, inevitably become hurt and harmful as an adult.

I used it with Gordon.

WHAT HAPPENED?

"Gordon," I said. "Think back to being about eight years old again. What did you have to do, how did you have to be, in order be psychologically safe?"

He thought. "Good, I had to be good, I had to be no bother, invisible almost, I had to be agreeable, I had to be quiet, I had to be obedient, I had to be controlled and I had to do my best."

I had written down on a notepad, "Good, no bother, agreeable, quiet, obedient, controlled, best."

I invited Gordon to look at those words, and then said, "What colour are those words?"

This always surprises patients. "Colour?" said Gordon, "what do you mean?"

I persisted, "Reading those words, what colour comes to mind?"

He paused, "Yellow"

"Any particular kind of yellow?"

"Yes, pale yellow."

"Okay, now Gordon think of you at your most distressed, say, for example, on that afternoon when you attempted to kill yourself, how did you feel, what feelings did you have?"

"Despair, useless, pathetic, weak, angry, hopeless, small, bad, disorganised."

"Now Gordon think of those words, what colour are they?"

"Black with red veins."

"Do you want them to go away?"

"Yes, yes, of course, I never want to feel like that again."

"Well, Gordon, in order to get rid of 'black with red veins,' you are going to have to stop being 'pale yellow.'"

He looked at me perplexed. I gently said, "Angry, hopeless, small, disorganised, useless, are the mirror opposites of good, doing my best, invisible, controlled, no bother, agreeable."

"How much are you an eight year old, pale yellow, at work?"

"All the time."

"And, in your relationships?"

"All the time."

"Now Gordon, there are strengths in pale yellow and in black with red veins. If you were to put those two colours together what colour would you have?"

"Persimmon," he said.

"Persimmon?" in ignorance, I queried.

"Yes, persimmon, you know burnt orange!" (Thanks Gordon.)

"Okay, Gordon, from now on you are going to go into the world as persimmon, no more pale yellow for you."

For the first time since I had met him he laughed.

"I am not sure everyone's going to like that," he said.

"Yes," I said, "it could be difficult being persimmon."

Giving up the psychological strategies you used to keep yourself safe as a child is always hard, but always necessary for recovery.

Delightfully, when I next visited Gordon he was wearing a dark orange tee shirt. He looked good in it.

I asked him, feeling as exhausted as he did, what a "persimmon person" would do about work.

He was on to it. "Take some time off?"

We quietly negotiated with his university. He was granted a six month sabbatical that was officially announced as a prize for his outstanding contribution to teaching. A few colleagues emailed him and congratulated him; said it was well merited. He was dismissive.

However, it may be that once a cognitive behaviourist, there is always a bit of CBT ready to be deployed.

I have three favourite CBT strategies for managing people with "depression," or "dependent personality disorder" or, as was really the issue in this case, a history of childhood neglect and abuse.

The first is especially for the desperate strivers like Gordon. When I first saw him in his house it was a mess. Mess clogs up our brain with visual distractions that increases cognitive load and reduces our working memory (such as our ability to keep multiple ideas in mind). As a consequence, the efficiency of our thinking is impaired. Mess is a drain on the brain.

So, I sat with him and said, "Now Gordon I have a new 'rule' for you that I want you, over the next month or so, to put into practice. And that is 'what's the *least* I can do today!'"

Needless to say Gordon was aghast. "No, not least, I must do more."

However, I persisted, "Go on, what's the *least* you could do today?

His house had an impressive view over an adjacent woodland and golf course. The house had been built to take advantage of the view with large, floor to ceiling, concertina windows built into the large back of the house family area. The only problem was the windows were filthy.

As I asked him, "What's the *least* you can do today" we were sitting looking at, but not out of, the dirty windows. After a couple of nudges, Gordon replied "Well, I could clean a window." There were, we counted, 144 individual windows inserted into his concertina doors.

"Okay" I said, "a window a day."

"Inside and out?" he asked.

"Only if you can manage it, but if it's too much do the inside first."

When I returned later that week he had cleaned the top three square windows inside and out. I congratulated him on his efforts. He dismissed my praise.

WHAT HAPPENED?

A week later he had cleaned fourteen windows and six weeks later the all the windows were crystal clean. He said, prophetically, "It's good to be able to see out."

After a month, Gordon was no longer on Avanza. Although he reported that his sleep had become disturbed and that he felt more agitated, there were two distinct benefits. One was that his agitation gave him more energy, and although a bit restless, he decided (with a nudge) it would be good to start to do some exercise.

My view is that with "depression," it is useful to decide when to hibernate and when to push oneself. Gordon noted that as a teenager and young man he had been a keen cyclist so went out and bought himself, (with his girlfriend's help) a new bicycle. His house was conveniently located near to a cycle path that took him down to a river and to literally a hundred kilometres of cycle pathways.

The other great benefit of being off Avanza was that slowly Gordon began to lose weight. When I first met him he was some twenty to twenty-five kilos overweight, which he found depressing and another reason to lambast himself. What noone had told him is that weight gain is a common side effect from taking Avanza, with about thirty percent of users gaining twenty to thirty kilos and a further twenty percent gaining ten to twenty kilos. I also noted that his weight gain was also likely to be Seroquel induced, because, again, weight gain from the use of "anti-psychotics" is very common.

In the event, Gordon also found coming off Seroquel relatively painless, albeit he had only been on it for about six months. There are well-recorded withdrawal effects from "anti-psychotics" and current best practice is that withdrawal from long-term "anti-psychotic" use is a very slow tapering of doses over one year.

We were now some three months post his suicide attempt and there were clear indications of improvement. Gordon and I met weekly for psychotherapy and he had monthly check-ins with his psychiatrist. Our psychotherapy sessions focussed on a core issue of his childhood. Gordon had an acute sense of not being enough, of being a burden, and spent his waking hours trying to anticipate and negate being found not enough or a burden.

He thus over-worked, over-prepared, over-did and took on responsibilities that he did not need to. He thus became ego depleted. Ego depletion is a useful working concept for people who have had childhoods like Gordon's.

Although introduced by Freud, ego depletion has been re-introduced into the psychology working parlance by motivational specialists such as Baumeister. Essentially, it can be shown that in order to function effectively, you need to match any energy outputs by restorative, energy inputs. Thus, if you are working hard and have other demands such as domestic and familial duties then these need to be offset by having time to one's self, good sleep and diet, and restorative time with friends and family members. It's really a question of looking at what drains away your energy and then what restores it to a good balance.

I invited Gordon to do my favourite ego depletion exercise. It goes like this.

I drew four large round circles on a piece of A4 paper.

I said, "Gordon, think about a typical week, when you were working, and I want you to think about how you used up your twelve 'energy eggs' that you have for each week. Energy eggs are markers of the amount of energy, both physical and psychological, that you put into each of these four baskets of your life."

Gordon looked at me a bit sceptically, but I continued.

"Okay, look at this first circle." I wrote the word WORK into that circle.

"Okay Gordon, think about it, how much physical and mental energy would you, in a typical week put into the work basket?"

Gordon paused, "I have twelve eggs?"

"Yes, but how many does it feel like you put into that work basket?"

"Ten."

In the next circle I wrote HOME.

"Now, Gordon, how many energy eggs does it feel like you put into your home life? Home includes all aspects of your home life, including things like paying bills, tidying up, doing maintenance, the washing, spending time with family members, etc."

"Three," said Gordon.

In the next circle I wrote RELATIONSHIPS.

"Okay Gordon, how much physical and psychological energy does it feel goes into your relationship with Amanda, your wife and your children?" (Gordon had two adult children living in Melbourne.) "How many eggs?"

"Four," said Gordon.

In the final circle I wrote SELF.

"Zero," said Gordon. (Oh Gordon, gotcha Gordon!)

I showed Gordon the result.

"So Gordon, in a typical week you put ten of your energy eggs into work, three into home, four into your relationships and none into you. That's seventeen energy eggs when you only have twelve. How does that feel?"

"It's totally out of balance," said Gordon reluctantly.

With clients who have had childhoods like Gordon's, this is nearly always the case.

"How does that feel?"

"Exhausting," said Gordon. He paused, "And I'm overdrawn. Every week I just get more exhausted."

He hesitated, "Why do I do that? Why do I over-perform, why do I try too hard?"

"Because," I said to Gordon, "approval is not love."

He looked at me as though I'd just slapped him very hard. He was totally taken aback.

"What do you mean?"

"I mean that because in your childhood you felt not enough, that you were not really lovable, you made yourself into a little pale yellow person in the hope that you would be approved of, but approval is not love, it's merely approval."

He still looked at me uncomprehendingly.

"Gordon," I said gently, "I love my children, but they are always doing things I disapprove of, and I love them for that too, but approval is not love. Your seventeen-energy-eggs-a-week life is impossible, it's exhausting, it's ego depleting, it's depressing and it's driven by your unconscious desire to get other people to approve of you. Yet really what you are seeking is that which you didn't get as a kid, which is love. Approval is not love."

Gordon looked at me wide eyed. "I never knew that."

Every now and then in therapy you have a moment that you just know is a breakthrough "aha" moment. This was one of those delightful occasions. We were on the way to recovery.

Then it all went horribly wrong.

Some three to four weeks earlier we had agreed that Gordon's dose of his serenic drug Lexapro would be reduced from 80mg (4 x 20mg tablets) to 60 mg a day. This was duly commenced.

I received a phone call early one morning from Amanda to say that Gordon was huddled up in the foetal position and sobbing that he wanted to die. He was shivering, sweating, was experiencing nonstop brain zaps and was extremely agitated; acute, "anti-depressant" withdrawal at its worst.

To be fair to the psychiatrist (and all of us), "anti-depressant" withdrawal (sorry, discontinuation syndrome in the nomenclature of the pharmaceutical companies), was at that time not well understood.

Lexapro was introduced in the early 2000s and by the time of Gordon's admission there was little clinical experience of withdrawing someone off Lexapro after long-term use. Long-term in Gordon's case was ten years of everyday nonstop use with, as he became increasingly tolerant to it, ever increasing doses.

I have always been intrigued that many psychiatrists can simultaneously believe that alcohol, cannabis, cocaine, ecstasy, heroin, dexamphetamine and methamphetamine cause tolerance, but their "psych meds" do not.

Anyone who drinks or smokes can recall that their first drinks or cigarettes caused them to be unwell. Yet with practice these adverse effects from inhaling or imbibing disappear.

Alcohol is a naturally occurring intoxicant. Fruit falls from trees into a puddle and ferments. Along comes a caveman who literally sees this watering hole, drinks the contents and becomes grossly intoxicated, then falls about and gets eaten by a sabre tooth tiger. This is clearly, in terms of survival, not helpful. So our brains "neuro-adapt" to any exposure to outside chemicals.

What happens is that from the first exposure to alcohol, the receptors on the cells in our brain affected by alcohol down cell regulate. They disappear back into the cell so that the individual has fewer receptors available, thus any incoming drug has less capacity to render the individual intoxicated. With practice, we become less affected by alcohol and every other drug we may elect to use.

This process for recreational drug use is well accepted. For example, in Alcohol Dependence Syndrome, which suddenly appeared as gospel in DSM III, the whole notion was that increased tolerance was the harbinger of heavier use, and as tolerance increased past a certain point, then withdrawal was, on any abrupt cessation, inevitable.

It is now clear that people experience withdrawal from "anti-depressants," yet the drug companies and most professionals refuse to accept that people become tolerant to them. Dr. Peter Breggin is a staunch supporter of the notion that "anti-depressants" cause tolerance. In a series of writings he has proposed that not only do long term users become tolerant to serenics, but such tolerance is itself a cause of relapse back into depression. The higher the dose rate, the more likely an individual is, on stopping "anti-depressant" use, to relapse into depression. Their brains have neuro-adapted to the point that there are not enough receptors left available to take up the levels of serotonin that an individual naturally creates.

Interestingly, this was exactly the argument that Prof. Griffith Edwards (the originator of the Alcohol Dependence Syndrome) made about alcohol dependent people relapsing. They quickly reinstated high levels of alcohol use because of their existing tolerance.

Mind you, like homosexuality, the valid, reliable, clinically proven concept of Alcohol Dependence Syndrome from DSM III and IV was, in DSM 5.0, suddenly gone. I almost miss it.

My experience is that long-term "anti-depressant" users get the worst of both worlds. Long-term use causes emotional blunting ("the land of blur") and then, if abstinence can be achieved, it can take ages for the brain to recover and put out enough receptors so that naturally occurring levels of serotonin can be enjoyed. So for many patients, it is an act of faith to believe that blur will eventually be replaced by any sense of wellbeing. Although it has to be acknowledged that immediately after totally ceasing use there can be a period of weeks (perhaps months) when blur is replaced by grrr, irritability and frustration until the brain recalibrates itself back to normal.

Nonetheless for Gordon, our lack of knowledge was very harmful. It was not an exaggeration to say he disintegrated. Following the phone call from his girlfriend, Gordon was taken to an Emergency Department where it was determined that Gordon was psychotic. He was placed back on Seroquel, on a much higher than previous dose, and three days later re-admitted to our hospital.

When I saw him he was highly agitated, frightened, bewildered and unfortunately but understandably, highly mistrusting of me and his doctor. To further complicate matters the psychiatrist who normally saw Gordon was away and the stand-in psychiatrist immediately put Gordon back on Avanza and upped his Lexapro back to the original 80 mg dose and declared, with conviction, that Gordon was "psychotically depressed."

Three steps forward, five back. When I next saw Gordon he was spikey, angry, wary, brittle and blaming. Why, he wanted to know, had we done this to him?

My position when things go wrong, as they will inevitably do, is to rely on and repair the therapeutic alliance. Therapeutic ruptures are part of doing psychotherapy and an important part. Understanding why a rupture has occurred is vitally important therapeutic information.

The key to understanding a therapeutic rupture is that from the therapist's perspective, it feels unfair. Here you are doing your best, but the patient has misconstrued your empathic, curious, loving, accepting, playful and skilled work, as being inimical to their wellbeing. There can be a little voice in your head that wants to tell the patient to fuck off, that their demands are bordering on entitlement. When this ripple of annoyance courses through you, I always translate entitlement into a small, young voice saying, "Please care for me, I'm helpless."

However, on the patient's side there is a sense of outrage. Traumatising childhoods make people vulnerable to the re-awakening of old wounds. I term this the trauma echo. Thus, there is in the current therapeutic rupture, an element of a wound from the past.

For Gordon, it became quickly apparent that he felt betrayed. His perspective was that he had put his faith in me, had trusted me and then, wham! I had metaphorically thrown him under a bus.

Managing a rupture is always about hearing and validating the perspective of the other and then together gently exploring the nature of the old, re-activated wound. It can be very hard work.

Much of my work with Gordon around his "not enough-ness" and his sense of being a burden had focussed on his relationship with his father. He said that his dad seldom had much to do with him. Gordon reported that his father was an intimidating character. On occasions his father took Gordon along to observe from a distance as he undertook life-saving heart surgery. Comments from other staff usually went along the lines of, "You must be very proud of your dad."

He was, but as Gordon and I agreed, that only emphasised to pale yellow little Gordon his belief of not measuring up.

However, it is often the parent that is not spoken about that is the most troublesome. So in this place of rupture I asked Gordon to talk to me about his mother. It took a while, but we got there in the end.

Gordon said that as a young child he had felt close to his mum and was sorry that his father treated her as "a servant." So, he tried as best he could to compensate for this and went out of his way to be helpful and considerate towards her.

I suddenly realised that he had developed his pale yellow persona for his mother.

Gordon reported that when he was ten he had developed asthma. Mild at first, it gradually worsened. He said that one day when he was twelve he was on the bus to school when his breathing became compromised. He also realised that he did not have his Ventolin inhaler with him. Upon arriving at school he used a nearby pay phone to call home, but his mum did not answer.

Because his breathing was becoming more laboured, he decided to catch the bus back home. On the bus his breathing became more and more difficult and he started to panic. He reported that the bus stop was some three hundred metres from his house and he said that with every step he thought he was not going to make it. On entering the house, he literally staggered into his bedroom to find his inhaler, but instead he found his mother in his bed with his father's brother.

The shock and bewilderment, plus his asthma, caused him to collapse. His mother called an ambulance. He described, that as the paramedics worked on him, he was terrified that he was going to die.

Two hours later when he had recovered sufficiently, his mother told him that if he ever said a word about what he had seen she would walk out of the house and never see him again. He never told. He still feels totally betrayed.

In the crisis of "serenic" withdrawal, this old deep dark wound was re-activated. The severity of his withdrawal was not just frightening, but like his asthma attack, physically challenging. I had put him in the place where an old wound was re-activated.

We slowly repaired the rupture and became more bonded because of it.

We agreed on a tapering regime for his Lexapro that became a template for many subsequent "anti-depressant" withdrawal exercises. It went as follows: day one 80mgs, day two 75mgs, day three 80mgs, day four 75mgs and up and down and so on for two weeks. Then day one 75mgs, day two 75mgs, day three 75mgs and so on for two weeks.

Then, day one 75 mgs, but day two 70mgs, day three 75mgs, day four 70mgs and so on. Then two weeks later down to 70mg a day for two weeks then another 5mgs every other day reduction.

It is telling that alcohol withdrawal can be completed safely in five days, heroin withdrawal can be completed in a week, and it is similar with methamphetamine and cannabis. But the safe withdrawal from psychopharmacological drugs can take ages.

It took Gordon two years.

In May 2019, The UK Royal College of Psychiatrists released an "anti-depressant" withdrawal warning statement. The British Daily Mail newspaper reported that doctors had been told to warn millions of their patients on the severity of "anti-depressant" side effects, often lasting for months. It was stated that although for years, health officials had played down withdrawal symptoms as "mild," the Royal College have now admitted the long-lasting severe symptoms that all patients should be made aware of when first prescribed.

This recognition is important even if it has not as yet been copied by other psychiatric associations worldwide. Indeed, there is now an established withdrawal protocol. Optimum best practice is currently deemed to be the conversion of whatever "anti-depressant" people are on to an equivalent dose of a liquid preparation of Prozac, the stabilisation of the patient on that dose (with the help, if necessary of a benzodiazepine to manage anxiety and panic attacks), and then reduction every two to four weeks in ten percent steps.

However, if all the above difficulties of side effects, sexual dysfunction, serotonin syndrome, the land of blur, grrr and withdrawal effects were not problematic enough there is now a developing literature that supports the idea that so-called "anti-depressants" have a very marginal, if any, clinical benefit. This re-evaluation of the effectiveness of serenics was driven by the pioneering work of Irving Kirsch (2002) who used American freedom of information legislation to gain access to drug companies' unpublished trials. His subsequent meta-analysis showed that although patients taking so-called anti-depressants had a significant reduction in reported depressive symptomatology, down 10 points on a well-regarded depression symptom scale, people in the placebo groups also had an eight point drop, so the difference between the two groups was of no actual clinical significance.

As David Healy (2016) has noted, this small difference may have been caused by the people in the active side of the trial experiencing side effects; so they knew they were on an anti-depressants. For a review of the current evidence read Richard Bentall's disturbing book *Doctoring the Mind* (2009) or Peter Gotzsche's recent review *Psychopharmacology is not evidence based medicine* in which he concluded, "I have come to the conclusion that anti-depressants should not be used by anyone and should be taken off the market."

However, there is a funny postscript to this case. I saw Gordon regularly over a four-year period and some five years after that I was walking through the centre of Singapore one evening when out of the front door of a very expensive hotel, stepped Gordon. It took both of us a minute to place each other, but when recognition had dually dawned, Gordon invited me for a drink.

As it happened I was in Singapore teaching about the management of alcohol and drug dependence for a local university's one-week extension course. It was a difficult gig. First, my accommodation was in a student hostel with no air conditioning. It was November so it was very hot and humid. The only transport option from my room to the lecture theatre was a twenty-five minute walk (impossible, I'd melt), or a ten minute trip in an un-airconditioned bus.

Also, because of the number of students enrolled in the course, I had to each day repeat the same lecture twice, in an inadequately air conditioned lecture theatre. Teaching and sweating is unpleasant. Furthermore, my audience was hard to engage with; the reserved cultural politeness was very different from what I normally experienced.

So, as I entered Gordon's hotel for a drink, I was impressed by the crisp cool air conditioning and the plush surroundings. Over drinks I caught up on Gordon's life. He had, without doubt, prospered. He was now a professor at a top five university, he and his wife were back living together and he was in Singapore on a five-day consultancy for a multi-national mining company.

He was staying in the hotel and he invited me for dinner in their five star restaurant. I remember we had great steaks and consumed, on Gordon's insistence, an extraordinarily expensive bottle of red wine.

I had during the course of dinner confided in Gordon that my current gig in Singapore was both hard work and not well renumerated. As it came time to settle the bill, Gordon said, "I'll pay, I have a very generous expenses allowance."

He then said, "Bill, I have to say it's very gratifying that I seem to be doing so much better than you."

Just in that moment, I wondered if pale yellow suited Gordon better.

Chapter Seven

The woman who drowned

Every now and then, a new patient turns up with whom you find yourself having an almost instant rapport. Emma was one such patient. She was referred by her GP for her 'alcoholism.'

I really dislike that term because it's pejorative and imprecise. It also prompts the use of the word 'alcoholic' - and I really don't like 'ic' words. They imply that the patient is just an alcoholic, a schizophrenic or a neurotic. Just as the word 'lunatic' is now pejorative, then so the other 'ic' words require removal from our clinical vocabulary. 'Ics' are also parents, children, friends, lovers, people with jobs, hopes and aspirations. Being labelled an 'ic' is one-dimensional, and there is also within the 'ics' a taint of biological determination and permanence.

"You're an alcoholic" misses the point. As a therapist, you always need to look beyond the substance and see what the psychological drivers were for that individual's over-reliance or dependence on alcohol. What happened to them to make them be like this? If you just focus on their 'alcoholism' you miss seeing the whole person and exploring with them the aetiology of their dependence.

Emma was a vivacious, forty-five year old, smart, funny, perfume retailer. I was immediately taken by her East London accent and, it has to said, her blue eyes, blonde hair and very fit appearance. I could easily imagine her being a very successful sales person. That she had a latent sexuality and a quick-witted flirty interpersonal style, made her even more likeable. I could see her being the ideal person to ask, "What perfume should I buy for my wife?"

My experience is that by the end of the first session you usually have a feel for how easy or difficult a patient is going to be to work with. I thought Emma was going to be easy. I actually have a four category assessment structure that assists me to gauge how I need to be with a particular patient and, for that matter, how hard I'll have to work.

Some patients (and Emma was one) are what I label the 'low positive regard' group. This group are the easiest to work with because they come into therapy with a capacity to trust the therapist and are open to making a connection. In contrast, the 'high positive regard group' can be very challenging. First conversations will often include a statement as to their excitement at being able to work with you, and an inference that they know you are just the person to help them. Unfortunately, "you are better than all the rest" (however, beguiling to hear) can quickly turn into you are a demon, a devil, a disappointment. It's all too easy to fall short.

Whenever I have a patient who is, at the outset, overblown in their praise of me, I quickly attempt to limit expectation. I also explore how 'let down' they have been in their past relationships. You need to be very alert to the potential for rupture and not fall into the heady trap of rescuing them from themselves.

The third group of patients are those with 'low negative regard.' These are the patients who come into therapy ready to grumble and find fault with you or your practice. Such patients will from the outset be censorious. They may complain about a whole host of matters from the parking, to the temperature of your room, the duration of their session or your fees. As can be appreciated, these patients are, in their interaction with you, telling you about their perspective on life. It is disappointing the world cannot be trusted, and they're constantly looking for the next adversity, the next let down. The need to be especially kind, especially considerate, to explore the disappointment of their being, to make an especially determined effort to establish a strong therapeutic relationship, is the absolute imperative in working with such patients.

Then the last group are the 'high negative regard' clients. Often coerced into therapy, they are disagreeable from the outset. They are quite upfront about the uselessness of therapy and can easily provoke in you a hostile counter-transference. In psychiatric nomenclature they are usually in the personality disordered domain. The key trick with such difficult patients is to realise from the off that they hurt too.

Their hostility is a defence; usually to avoid connection. I always remind myself when becoming irritated by their demeanour that 'being difficult' is about complexity. A social worker I was supervising perspicaciously remarked, "Ha, yes Bill, if you call them difficult it makes them into a wall, but if you see them as complex then they are a maze." Um, wish I'd said that. So, I have always encouraged my colleagues to delete the word difficult and replace it with complex.

Emma's response to my "What brings you to see a psychologist?" opening question brought a very frank response.

"Bill, I'm a total fuck up, a walking nightmare, a train wreck."

Her words were at total odds with her appearance.

WHAT HAPPENED?

"Really?"

"Yes, really."

"Okay, tell me about it."

And she did, and I could see why she thought that she was a fuck up.

Emma reported that she grew up in West Ham in London and her father, a car mechanic, left her mother (a nurse) when she was very young, about three. Her mother then juggled being a nurse and being a mum, so Emma recalled often being shunted off to relatives and day care. She recalled that her mother had a couple of subsequent relationships, but none of them were long lasting. She said that she did okay at school, but was never a stand-out student. However, she was good at sport, especially netball. She was also a runner, having, in her early twenties, completed the London marathon a couple of times. She said that apart from never seeing her dad, her childhood was unremarkable. She emigrated to Australia with her first husband when she was twenty-four, but he left her when she was thirty.

Given the 'alcoholism' referral, I asked, "How much, if anything at all, did your drinking have to do with your divorce?"

Emma quickly replied, "One hundred percent. I told you I was a fuck up."

My position with any form of drug dependence is always to remember that lots of people use drugs, but only a minority become dependent. With alcohol, out of all the people who drink, about ten percent become dependent. With cannabis, it's about five percent, LSD less than one percent, XTC about the same. Even with the so called 'most addictive drugs in the world,' the rates for cocaine are about ten per cent, opiates and the stimulants (such as methamphetamine) no more than a fifth.

The message of this is that most drug users do not become dependent. An interesting question is why not? The answer is they don't need to. Recreational, non-dependent users use substances to enhance their lives, to have more fun. Their use is just an add on. A glass of red wine with a steak, an XTC tab at a gig or dexies to improve essay writing make the world go a bit better.

However, dependent users use substances to improve how they feel. They discover, usually in adolescence, that substances soothe. Whereas non-dependent users can self-soothe (by talking to a parent, friend or partner), dependent users are driven by the need to blot out how they feel. They thus become reliant upon the drug to manage their emotions. Unfortunately, such use is merely an emotional detour. Next day the pain is back so another fix is required. As this reliance increases then so does the emotional pain.

Being dependent also brings its own sense of failure. No one ever sets out to become drug dependent, but having arrived there, the realisation of 'I'm hooked,' 'I can't do without,' increases the underlying emotional distress that got them dependent in the first place. The issue with substance dependence is always to look beyond the substance and find what lies underneath. What happened to them?

It is usually childhood neglect and/or sexual abuse. Some years ago a medical colleague and I reflected on the prevalence of childhood sexual abuse in our cohort of female patients. He estimated about seventy percent and I thought possibly eighty percent. I duly pulled the case notes of the last fifty female patients whom we had admitted. We were both wrong. The figure was one hundred percent.

So I was intrigued by Emma. I explored with her the likelihood of her being sexually abused. She was adamant that nothing untoward had ever happened.

Her utmost issue was not her past, but her present. She informed me that she was in a Family Court tussle with her ex over the children. She had two children to two different fathers. The first, a boy, now seventeen, was from her first marriage and the second from a second relationship. But, the ex she was contesting custody with was not the father of either child.

As I teased out her complicated relational history she reiterated, "See, I'm a nightmare. I get into relationships and then I fuck them up by drinking."

Patients with Family Court issues always pose a risk, and that is to do with confidentiality. It's all very well trotting out the standard "Whatever is said in this room remains in this room," but my experience with Family Court matters is that it is just not true. The other side always subpoenas the notes. In order to protect my client I warn them at the outset of the likelihood that my notes will be subpoenaed. This always causes distress. What of the affair/my drinking/the illegitimate child/the one million dollars in my secret overseas bank account?

I always reassure them and say, "I will write your notes from the perspective of them being seen by your ex. I will omit to write anything you believe to be detrimental to yourself. I will include any hostile, malfeasant, nasty, or criminal actions that you report to me about your ex. If you wish, you may at the beginning of each session, see my notes from the session before."

My experience of doing this is that it reassures the client as to their confidentiality and that I am on their side. It is vital, especially when dealing with messy divorces, to be able to get your client into a place of honest reflection. My position is that the disharmony, the rupture, is not his or her fault; it is both of them - one hundred percent.

With Emma there was, of course, the issue of her drinking. As I noted to her, I needed to include reference to this in my notes. But as I pointed out, it was not as though her ex was unaware of it. My position on such things is always to write, where possible, of gains (such as days sober, improved liver function, better personal relationships), rather than focus too much on lapses or scandalous binges.

WHAT HAPPENED?

Emma's current dilemma was that the Family Court had established an interim order in which she could only see her children under supervision. The order thus gave the ex (non-biological father) full-time custody of her children. The Court had determined this largely because some three months prior Emma had collected the children from school for one of her informally agreed three nights a week of shared custody, and on the way home had been involved in a significant road traffic accident. As it happened it was not her fault. She was hit by another motorist who had ignored a red light. The trouble was, when the police arrived, they breathalysed both drivers. The 'at fault' motorist was sober, Emma was not. She had to telephone her ex in order for him to look after the children while she was processed.

The next day, he applied for a court order that in due course gave him interim full custody. Emma said she was devastated.

I asked her my usual motivational assessment questions. As one of my former colleagues once, very insightfully, said, "Motivation is not stuff you can put into people. They have to find it for themselves."

Over the years of working with dependent drug users I have developed what I have found to be a very useful and informative motivational screening test. It is comprised of three questions.

"Emma," I said, "on a zero to ten scale, with zero being not at all and ten being lots, how much is your drinking a problem for you?"

Emma instantly said, "Ten out of ten."

The above question is useful in two ways. It is very logical; how does the client rate their problem. Second, it is a reflection of the impact their drinking has on them. It's not about the impact on others. My view is that drug use starts being problematic for the user when they start to consider doing something about it.

My second question was:

"Emma, on a zero to ten scale, with zero being not at all and ten being lots, how much are you concerned about your drinking?"

Emma was there in a flash, "Ten out of ten."

This second question is telling. People can have a problem and not be at all concerned about it. I once used these questions (they are good with any motivational issue) with a severely diabetic woman. She noted that her diabetes was a 'ten out of ten' problem, but when asked how concerned she was about her diabetes she replied quite simply, "Naught out of ten … I want to die."

The other trick is that the question is about concern. It is an emotional question. My experience is that significant behaviour change is much more driven by emotion than logic. Especially with alcohol and drug dependence, logic is not enough.

However, the third question is the killer - a gotcha question.

"Emma, on a zero to ten scale how much do you desire to be abstinent from alcohol, totally sober, for the next three years?

Emma instantly responded, "Ten out of ten."

"Okay," I said, "let's do it."

Desire is very important. It is a better predictor of what people will do than their *belief* in their capacity to do it (so-called self-efficacy).

I worked with Emma over the next six months. My intervention was my standard managing alcohol dependence paradigm. That is, get sober first then address the underlying issue that drove the individual into dependence.

In this process it's important to have a purpose. This is never more so than giving up something one has loved and has relied upon. Thus, giving up alcohol to be sober doesn't in my view work. It's a bit like running every day to get fit. My personal experience is that I only run every day because there is a fun run to do some three months down the track. (And, I need, of course, to still beat my daughters).

With Emma that purpose was easily identified.

When I said, "Emma, what's the purpose of being sober?"

She instantly said, "To get the kids back."

Priority is everything. I held my hands out. "Emma," I turned my left palm up. "This hand is alcohol."

I turned over my other hand. "Emma, this is your children. Which hand matters most?"

She quietly said, "The right hand, my kids."

Then, "Emma, is your drinking worth it?"

"No, no, no."

"Emma, if you drink can you win?"

"No."

"So Emma, what are you going to do?"

"I'm going to stop drinking."

"Because?" (Because is a lovely word. If you ask 'why' you will get a logical response, but 'because' always prompts a more 'feelings' reply. If bold you can use three, maybe four, in a row and go deeper each time).

"Because I want my kids back."

"Because?"

"Because I want to show them I'm a good mum."

"Because?"

"Because," she gulped, and held back tears.

"Because, Bill, I'm better than this." (Gotcha!)

I then remember doing something I only do occasionally, and always carefully.

My office has an outside balcony that looks over an adjacent house and a side street.

I said to Emma, "I want you to go outside and shout at the top of your voice, 'I don't fucking drink!' I want the whole neighbourhood to hear you. I want you to shout it out over the roof tops."

She stared at me. She was clearly tempted to say 'no way.' She gritted her teeth. She went out, and in the middle of a balmy summer afternoon, she shouted out so the whole neighbourhood could hear.

"I don't fucking drink! I don't fucking drink. I don't fucking drink. I don't fucking drink. I don't fucking drink. I don't fucking drink. I don't fucking drink."

Delightfully, a man passing by stopped and listened and then when Emma had finished said, "Well done girl, I wish I could say that."

Emma came back in, tears were coursing down her face; she stood in front of me.

"Thank you," she said. She paused, smiled, and said very deliberately, "Bill, I don't fucking drink."

All went well. She got to ninety days sober (always a milestone). She carefully started a new relationship. She got a different, better paid job. She got to 180 and the ex relented and allowed her (despite the court order) to pick up the kids from school and have them over for dinner. She got to 275 days. The new boyfriend asked her to marry him.

We went back to Family Court and in the foyer before the hearing, the ex agreed to give her some cash (they had lived together for five years in a house to which both had contributed). It was also agreed that Emma could have the kids three nights a week. The only stipulation was that when she was in charge of the kids she had to be totally sober.

The Family Court agreed to what had been agreed in the foyer. I left the court that day thinking, "what a good outcome." Emma was jubilant. She stood in the foyer of the court chatting to her two children. Even the ex and the fiancé shook hands. I left feeling job well done; that's it.

But it wasn't.

I walked into my office some nine months later to be warned by our practice manager that she had put someone in my room who said she was a former patient, but wouldn't give her name. She said the unknown patient was in a terrible state.

It was Emma. The practice manager had understated her presentation. Emma was drunk. She had two black eyes, she was wearing scruffy clothes and she was sobbing. "Bill," she slurred, "I'm a fuck up, I'm a nightmare, I want to die."

Fortunately for me (and Emma) at the time, I was not only a Clinical Psychologist in a private practice, but due to a strange confluence of circumstances, I was also a Director of a private psychiatric hospital that managed co-occurring mental health and drug dependence issues. I rang Dr. John, the very man who had inveigled me into getting involved in the hospital.

"Ah, Dr. John. I have a problem."

The hospital was literally down the road; he came, he admitted Emma on the spot, and then he sobered her up.

It's very satisfying to be able to provide instant, wrap-around care.

It takes about four days for people who have been on a bender to feel well again. Ten milligrams of Valium four times a day also helps. A few days later I went down to the inpatient unit. Emma was sitting in her room crying. I have a standard phrase for patients who have relapsed and who are re-admitted.

I said, "Emma, it's really good to see you again. But I'm really sorry about the circumstances of our meeting. Do you want to tell me what happened?"

She looked at me. She was totally defeated. "Bill, I did it again, I fucked up, everything was going so well. I had everything, and now I have nothing."

The story came out haltingly.

Following the Family Court case she had moved in with her fiancé, but as a security she had used the money she had received in the settlement to buy herself a small town house that was close to her kid's school. On the days that were her days with the kids she stayed at the townhouse. She and the fiancé were planning their marriage. She had also left her old job and had started working in a managerial capacity for the fiancé in his business equipment firm. Emma noted that, "I had the kids, I had a house, I had money in the bank, I had my best ever job and I was about to marry the best man ever - and I fucked it up!"

"So Emma," I queried. "How did you fuck it up?"

"Easy," she said. "One night when the kids were over, I must have been about eighteen months or a bit more sober. We were eating their favourite, spaghetti bolognaise, so I went to the fridge and opened a bottle of vodka I had put in the fridge that morning and over the next hour I drank it. I think I collapsed on the floor. The kids called the ex and he now has them full-time. I got into a terrible fight with my fiancé, I've lost my job and then I got drunk in a hotel and some guy punched me."

"Yes," I said, "your black eyes are spectacular." She smiled ruefully.

"Emma, look, I always knew that we never really got to the bottom of your drinking. While you're in here, and I suspect that we'll keep you for a week or so more, I want to explore what happened to you to make you be like this."

"What do you mean? What makes me a fuck up?"

"Not quite, I want to explore what makes you fuck up. That's different to *being* a fuck up."

WHAT HAPPENED?

She just looked at me bleakly. "Okay, if you say so."

Being self-destructive is a fascinating psychological defence. On the surface it defies belief. It just doesn't make sense. However, there's always, underneath, a reason. The trick of managing a patient as blatantly self-destructive as Emma is not to engage in logic.

There is always the temptation to tell the patient that if they do X again then Y will follow. However, the earnest instruction not to self-destruct is merely pointing out what the client already knows. It can fuel the very deployment of the self-destructive behaviours the keen therapist is warning about.

Whenever tempted to cry, "Can't you see what you are doing to yourself?" I take a step back and be quiet. Of course they can see what they are doing and that is why they do it.

So 'mind detective' is where to go. Explore together why self-destruction works. What does self-destruction protect the patient from?

Oh, and of course, go back to childhood.

So a few days later, I broke all the rules about time boundaries and deliberately allowed myself to have a double session with Emma. I am a stickler for the fifty minute session. I train my patients up for it. I start my patients on time, usually on the hour, but the fifty minutes are carefully orchestrated. I know that at about forty minutes into the session I will say in a suitable pause, "I'm really sorry Freda, but our time today is almost up." That is a flag. As the fifty minutes arrives I say, "Sorry Freda, we must end here for today." Some patients resist and want a bit more. But I'm always more determined than they are. (I often have another patient on the hour so I must not be late). I say, "Freda, can you talk to Jennifer our secretary and make another appointment so we can continue our work?" If necessary, I stand up. I finish every session with, "Thank you for coming today, take care."

Just to assist the process, I have two clocks. One the patient can see and one I can see. Interestingly, once the patients have learned the time rules I often spot them checking the clock to see how to manage the remaining time. I confess that the clock visible to the patient is always two minutes ahead of time.

So I went down to the hospital, found Emma and then walked with her back to my office. As noted, my office at the time was about 150 metres from the hospital. Seeing patients while they are sitting in or on a bed is never desirable. Therapy needs to be done face to face, and literally on the same level. Also for many traumatised patients, having a male in their bedroom is threatening and unsafe.

I am very cautious when walking a patient from A to B. Very early on in my career I was asked to see a young man who had had a very bad LSD trip. The first time I saw him he was highly agitated and disorganised. It was hard to reassure him he was safe. Additionally, he didn't like (who would?) being detained in a locked ward.

A few days later, I saw him again. He was much improved, although still uncertain as to whether the hallucinations he had experienced were real. Nonetheless, he still engaged well with me. As the session concluded he asked if he might be allowed out of the ward. It was a cool, but sunny winter's day. The hospital, being an old asylum, had delightful grounds. I duly spoke to the nursing staff about his request and left the ward. Two hours later, albeit with an escort, he managed to run in front of a bus and kill himself.

I have, ever since, when placed in the position of walking anywhere with an inpatient, been a very observant escort.

I sat Emma down. My "How's your world?" question was met with a shrug.

"Ah," I said, "feeling shit, eh?"

Empathic conjecture is a useful way of making connection with a patient. Especially one who is struggling, and you don't even have to get it right. A 'feelings statement' allows the patient to feel your empathy.

Emma said, "Look, I'm less bad. Derek," (the ex) "brought the children in last night and I'm going to be allowed home for the weekend, so I guess it's start again time."

I said, "Yes, that's what I'd like to explore. Do you know, Emma, you said on your very first meeting that you were a fuck up. Remember?"

"Oh yes, I say that all the time."

"Well, I owe you an apology. You know I've never really explored with you about why you fuck things up. So I'd like to do that today."

"Oh," she said. "I think that's just me."

"Emma, today I'd like to explore the underlying reasons for you electing, on occasions, to fuck up. I think that's very different from being a fuck up."

This blurring of 'what I do' into 'who I am' is a classic marker of shame. "You're a bad girl for hitting your brother," type statement is the beginning of such blurring. The statement, "I love you, but sometimes your behaviour is disappointing," keeps the distinction between what you do and who you are.

"So Emma, let's explore why you self-destruct. Go back to your childhood. Let's review that."

I got her to recall her early years in London, describe the house she lived in, talked about dad's desertion and then her life with mum. Still suspicious about the possibility of sexual abuse, I explored her mother's relationships with men, her experience of males and male school teachers. There was literally nothing of note.

We moved into the second hour.

I asked her to give me a feel for a typical day when she was going to primary school. She talked happily about her early experiences, her early friendships. She started to talk about her best friend, Sally, whom she had recently re-connected with via Facebook. She talked about them recalling playing in the park up the road, the long British summer nights.

And suddenly she stopped. She checked herself. I saw her body tense.

Her voice changed. Her accent became more pronounced. She started speaking directly to the floor. She said, in a sing-song, six or seven-year-old voice;

"I loved playing with Sally. She lived two doors up. There was a park. In summer we'd all meet up. There were lots of local kids, we'd take our dolls, it was fun. It was fun."

"Mum had one rule, I didn't like it. Mum used to say be home at six for a bath. I didn't like it. I had to stop playing with Sally. I had to run home. I had to be ready for bath. I didn't like it. I had to run it myself. I had to be careful. Not too hot, not too cold. Mum would then come. Wash my hair. Bathe me."

Emma went very quiet. She said in a low, very small voice, "Sometimes she drowned me."

My usual impassive poker face didn't stand a chance.

Incredulously, I said, "Sorry what did you say? Your mother drowned you?"

I saw Emma shiver. She was shaking. She was crying, saliva was dribbling from her mouth, mucous ran from her nose. She was ghostly white.

"Yes, I hear doors slam. I don't like it. She runs into bathroom. Hold me underwater. There was nothing I could do. She was too strong. Too big, too strong. I'd go away."

She was shaking, there were goosebumps on the skin on her arms. Tears were pouring down her face, running into her nasal mucous and streams of saliva.

Reeling, I asked the only stupid, obvious question my bewildered mind could manage.

"But, you're alive?"

"Oh yes," said Emma. "She kill me, she save me. She a nurse. Wake up in bed all wet. Wake up in bed naked. It was summer. I didn't like it. No, no, no, I didn't like it."

I removed a towel that was fortuitously in the sports bag under my desk. I dried her eyes, wiped away the mucous and the saliva. I laid her on the sofa and covered her with a blanket; she fell asleep.

I sat with her. Some twenty minutes or so later, she stirred.

She said, "I've never told anyone about that. I wonder if it's true. I think she may have done it about a dozen times. It was always in summer."

I got Emma a cup of tea. I told her that I believed her. I told her it was not her fault. I told her I admired her. I told her that what had happened to her was unconscionable.

I told that self-destruction was always better than allowing someone else to shoot you down. That, if when a child everything is going good and somebody comes along and destroys you, then, as an adult, when things become good, you will destroy it yourself.

We sat and cried together.

She was discharged three days later. She said, "I don't think I need to see you again."

I didn't agree. I thought we were at the beginning of a new journey, but I said, "You know where I am."

She never came to see me again.

Some years later, walking through a shopping centre, we literally walked into each other. "Emma!" I said "How are you?"

She smiled and in a very loud voice shouted, "I don't fucking drink!"

People stopped to look. I am sure they couldn't understand why we were laughing.

Chapter Eight
Perfect psychosis

I first met Georgia in group. I was immediately touched by her warm engagement and her acceptance of her fellow participants; especially those who had the most complex and difficult childhoods. She oozed empathy and was completely accepting of the idiosyncrasies, the follies, even the most self-destructive of acts of her fellow group members.

In her late twenties, she was an attractive, funny, clever, overweight woman. Despite her warm, usually smiling disposition, her eyes spoke volumes about her past. Her eyes were desperate, full of pain, doubt, pleading and wariness. She had a fragile presence.

Despite her very evident compassion for others it quickly became evident in group that she was very self-critical and self-blaming. Her generosity, her acceptance, her empathy and warm curiosity only extended to the other.

She was a classic case of the "trauma split," totally accepting that what had happened to the other group participants was not their fault, but sure that she was totally responsible for what had occurred to her. She was guilty, she had brought this on herself; everything was her fault. She reeked of self-loathing.

Georgia said that she had a "schizo-affective" disorder and had also been diagnosed as having "bipolar." She said she was on "a shit load of meds," that included "anti-psychotics," an "anti-depressant" and a "mood stabilizer."

Over several groups, her history came out: the "what happened to her," was a history of shocking sexual abuse, secrets, and the lies of a "perfect family."

Georgia asked if we could "do some one on ones?" and I readily agreed as I felt there was a lot that was not being talked about, so individual psychotherapy was an opportunity to explore and discover what had really happened.

We started with an exploration of her family. Over several sessions it gradually transpired that her childhood was a very complex marinade of toxicity overlaid with perfection.

Her father was a very successful corporate lawyer. Georgia noted that his personality, detached, particular, unemotional, demanding, authoritarian, aloof, pedantic and literal, fitted the corporate world perfectly. He was very good at what he did.

As he prospered, the family prospered. Georgia's childhood home was a mansion in the most select of suburbs. Her suburb was on a peninsular by a river. She said she had grown up in "a sort of gated community for the very wealthy," that few people from elsewhere ever visited.

She recalled that as a child, every summer was endless days of playing with her peers from similar wealthy families. Because the traffic into and around the peninsular was only local residents she and her peers were allowed to roam free. There was swimming, kayaking, fishing, cycling, playing street cricket, hide and seek, or just hanging out in the parks and gardens of their manicured and exclusive idyllic retreat.

At home the perfection continued. Not only was the house immaculate and exclusive, but the walls were adorned with happy family pictures of her and her sisters, her mum and dad all prospering, all being happy, all being successful: the perfect family.

However, beneath the veneer of total upper class awe and respectability there were demons. Most particularly her father, whose personality was not suited to parenting or domesticity, and her mother, ostensibly a kind woman, who was in thrall to her father.

Georgia reported that she and her sisters were really "just tokens" of her parents' perfectness. When her father was due home from work, all the toys, mess, and real life, would literally be swept under the carpet and thus, beautiful clean sanitised order was restored.

The only time Georgia really saw her father was at dinner, a time of "no elbows on the table" and "pleases and thank yous" and "eat up all your food" and "sit up straight" and "don't talk with your mouth full." Her father's word and thoughts were the law. She reported that aged about eleven and irritated by the behaviour of one of her sisters, she had sworn. Dad ordered mum to "wash her mouth out with soap," which was duly done.

Georgia reported that at the local primary school she had been perfect. She was both academically talented and athletic (a sprinter), she duly excelled. In her last year at primary school she was a prefect. She was also good at drama and singing, so at the end of year dramatic productions, she was centre stage. More photographs for the house wall of fame. Georgia noted that she did everything that was expected of her. She was, she wryly noted, "the token that delivered perfection for the perfect family."

Yet Georgia knew the perfection was only a veneer. Underneath there was nothing solid; a confusing amalgam of all; but nothing. Her relationship with her mother was tenuous, so obviously second to her mother's relationship to her father. Her relationship with her dad was non-existent. Georgia confessed that when aged about nine or ten she constantly fantasised about her parents getting divorced so then dad *would have* to spend time with her at the weekends.

There is considerable research literature about "high expressed emotion" families and their psychological impact. The characteristics of Georgia's family, with its acute, but unspoken tension between the father, mother and children, coupled with the highly critical even hostile nature of her father with his over-investment in "success," plus very little parental warmth and low positive tone, have all been demonstrated to be "schizophrenogenic." One can imagine Georgia's confusion at the ongoing perpetuated falsehood of "on the surface perfection," while underneath there was nothing.

Being perfect is, of course, hard work. This is especially so when being perfect is still not enough to get you what you want; which is connection, a sense that you matter, a sense of being special, a sense of being loved.

Georgia told her story. She was perceptive and insightful. Such lack of connection in this ostensibly perfect home made her vulnerable to much less perfect attention from elsewhere, especially when posing as connection and acceptance.

It unfortunately, perhaps inevitably, duly appeared.

Craig was the son of one of the other families in the lovely gated community. Five years older than Georgia, Craig was an awkward child, an odd misfit. It is easy to envisage a somewhat out of place Georgia being drawn towards a similarly displaced, not quite right, older child who paid her attention. Georgia reported that when she was eight or nine and playing with her girl gang, Craig often hung around the edges, circling around on his battered green bike.

I asked what happened. Georgia acknowledged, in classic trauma style, that she could only report on what had happened if she told the story as though it had happened to someone else. Known as "low narrative," Georgia told that in the summer when she was nine she had been playing cricket and then much to her annoyance she had been bowled out.

Georgia reported that she was sitting under a tree, and still annoyed about her dismissal, when she was approached by Craig. At first he taunted her about getting out, but then invited her to have a ride with him on his bike. Georgia said that he pedalled her to a secluded part of the river where there was a diving platform. Here he told her to lie down and then proceeded to give her instructions. These involved her slowly undressing and allowing Craig to stroke and touch her body.

Georgia reported that in her perfect family, sex was never mentioned. It was a taboo subject. She never saw her parents be sexual or affectionate, so she literally knew almost nothing about sex. Georgia reported that Craig's attention, his excitement, his interest was weird, but she liked it. Georgia reported that over that summer these episodes of "being told what to do" by Craig occurred with increasing frequency.

Georgia also reported that as the summer progressed Craig became more and more obsessed with her, which for her was beguiling. Although there was a bit of her that knew what was occurring was weird and wrong, she enjoyed the connection with Craig. It was good being special, being pursued, being wanted.

Georgia reported that the end of summer and the return to school naturally reduced their contact. However, Craig would on occasions follow her on his bike and she also sometimes found him watching her.

Georgia said that the following summer Craig's interest and attention were quickly re-instated; as were the instructions. Physically advanced for her age, these instructions eventually included being told to allow him to have penetrative sex with her, which she did, after which Craig became increasingly controlling and demanding. This continued unabated for the next two years. Georgia noted that she knew that what was happening was unusual and wrong, yet Craig's on-going surveillance of her, his obsession with her, his stalking of her and his increasing aggression made her believe that she had no choice, but to do what she was told.

Georgia reported that the transition from her primary school to a prestigious private girls' school resulted in "things spiralling out of control."

First, Craig had obtained a driving licence and then a car. He became even more demanding, leaving empty flower pots on the wall of her house to indicate that he expected her to climb out of her bedroom window at night and meet him to go for a drive and have sex.

He also gave her a mobile phone so that he knew where she was at all times. His sexual behaviour became increasingly unpleasant and involved degrading and humiliating bondage and sadomasochistic behaviour. Resistance seemed impossible; Craig became violent if thwarted.

The ignition to this explosive keg occurred when Georgia, aged thirteen, confided to one of her friends that she was concerned she may be pregnant. This confidential conversation spread like wildfire through the school and eventually Georgia was summoned to a meeting with the chaplain.

Although Georgia managed to initially deny any "wrong doing," word of her "ignominy" also reached the local private boys school, where Craig was a final year student. He accosted Georgia on her way home from school and in a rage broke her finger.

WHAT HAPPENED?

Georgia went home and said she had fallen over.

Georgia noted that as all this was unfolding, she became concerned that Craig was out to get her. She became increasing aware of him stalking her as she went to and from school. She began to have thoughts that he was spying on her via the mobile phone he had given her. Had he hacked her computer?

As Georgia became increasing distressed and terrified, she discovered that if she picked the skin on her fingers the pain would somehow soothe her. This slowly graduated into cutting her arms which, although painful for the moment, brought her relief from her increasingly troubled and scary thoughts.

Georgia was then called into a meeting at school that involved the principal and her parents. Her increasingly poor academic record, her at times odd behaviour, her emotional outbursts, her occasional non-attendance were all reviewed. The previously perfect child was letting her perfect family down.

It is often very disheartening (but often very informative) to have an adult survivor of childhood sexual abuse tell their "unaware" parents what had happened to them. It is disheartening because the adult response to the new information is often so inadequate, so off the mark, that you despair for the child. However, you can be instantly informed as to why the sexual abuse occurred.

One client, referred for "chronic depression," gradually, hesitantly, told of being raped from the age of ten to fourteen by her much older brother. She could not understand why it had happened. Was it her fault? Had she encouraged it? She had never told a soul and only indirectly alluded to her abuse by writing me a letter in which she made oblique references to "family trouble."

My stance is that the best antidote to shame is to face it head on and bring a cleansing searchlight of truth to the matter.

This client, a very successful and high ranking university academic, was not convinced. However, over time as our work together emboldened her (as she trusted me more), she eventually agreed to tell her parents what had happened to her. Her parents lived in a different state so she booked a flight for what she called "the big weekend of truth."

On her return I asked, "How's your world?"

Her reply was "It now has clarity."

She reported that she had sat her parents down at the dining room table and said, "I have something to tell you."

Her mother said, excitedly, "Oh, are you coming back to live here?"

"No, I'm not," she said, "what I want to say, and it is hard for me to do so, is that for a five-year period Allan used to force me to have sex with him."

Her mother replied by saying, "Ah, I wondered why you never seemed to get on as well with Allan as your other brothers. Hey, I have an idea. Why don't you bring your family over at Christmas and we'll have a big dinner and we can all be friends again?"

The patient reported that the total inadequacy of the response was liberating. Her emancipation was further enhanced when her father said, "Well, I guess worse things happen." He then excused himself to do some gardening.

The patient noted that it dawned on her, there and then, that her brother had realised the inadequacy of their parents, and the very poor connection in the family, so he knew he could literally get away with raping her.

My client said she left the house smiling, walked to a nearby restaurant and spent the evening telling a complete stranger the story she had never dared speak about. The client noted that she had realised, "It was not my fault."

Unfortunately, such disclosures are not always as cathartic. Jessica, who was nineteen, was referred to me for her "methamphetamine dependence."

It quickly transpired that she had, from the age of seven until about fourteen, been repeatedly sexually abused by an uncle. Despite telling her parents she didn't like him, she was regularly dropped off at his house for sleepovers or, on a couple of occasions, for several weeks at a time when her parents went on holiday without her.

As is often the case, sexual abuse in childhood results in further sexual abuse. The damning evidence is that the best predictor of being sexually abused as an adult is to be sexually abused as a child. Although counter-intuitive, the fact is, if you are not protected from sexual abuse as a child, you fail to learn how to protect yourself as an adult. Thus, you do not keep yourself safe.

There is a chilling piece of research that unfortunately demonstrates this only too well. Twenty-five women, who had been sexually abused as children, were matched to twenty-five peers who had not been so abused.

Each participant was shown a video tape of three young women, around twenty years old, getting ready to go out for a night. All the participants were told that if at any time they thought something in the video was untoward, then they needed to click the remote and stop the video.

The video showed the women walking into a bar and getting drinks. At some stage they were approached by three men, one of whom knew one of the girls. The video then showed one of the men offering to buy one of the girls a drink. In so doing he moved her away from her friends. They were depicted talking animatedly and then the male offered to buy her another drink. However, he told her that he needed to go to an ATM to get some cash.

He then asked her to accompany him to the ATM, but on the way suggested that rather than going back to the bar, "why didn't she come with him and have a drink with him at his place?" She agreed and after having further drinks at his place, she was raped.

WHAT HAPPENED?

What is fascinating about this research is that *all* of the women who had *not* been sexually abused, stopped the tape somewhere between the woman being offered a drink away from her friends, or when invited out of the bar.

None of the women who had been sexually abused as children stopped the tape. When de-briefed these respondents all stated something along the lines of "He seemed nice I felt it would be wrong to say no or upset him."

What keeps you safe as a child (that often means going along with the predator), becomes very unhelpful and harmful as an adult.

This was exactly the scenario with Jessica. When males paid her attention, she frequently ended up having sex with them, because even though she didn't want to, she also did not want to upset them. Such males included one of her school teachers and the school chaplain.

I was present when Jessica told her parents about being raped by her uncle. It was an event that has stayed with me because of the totally appalling reaction by her parents. Her mother, on hearing Jessica hesitantly and anxiously tell of being raped, looked at the floor and said absolutely nothing. She did not move.

Her father said, "Well, what about your drug use, that's the real problem, isn't it? Are you going to stop?"

Bewildered, Jessica said, "Yes,, Dad."

And that was it. Her parents then stood up and left my office.

Her parents' response told volumes about Jessica's childhood of neglect. A mother who totally lacked the capacity to empathise or attune to her daughter's needs, coupled with an emotionally avoidant, authoritarian father, were the (unwitting) architects of Jessica's sexual abuse and then compensatory drug dependence.

She didn't stop her drug use, and sadly died from a drug overdose some two years later. I suspect that she had nothing to live for, indeed never had anything to really live for, but after that day, I totally understood why Jessica took refuge in alcohol, sex and methamphetamine.

Such cases tend to confirm Jean-Paul Satre's gloomy prognosis: "One is never finished with one's family, it's like the smallpox that catches you as a child and leaves you marked for life."

In my work with her, Georgia was adamant that she was in no way going to tell her parents the truth. The reason being, that when aged about thirteen, she was sufficiently distressed, after being raped yet again, to have attracted her mother's interest when she arrived home. Haltingly, Georgia confessed to the fact that she had been out with Craig and he had raped her.

Her parents' response was to see this as a "one-off" and convey to Georgia the idea that because Craig had "learning difficulties" perhaps he didn't understand the true nature of what he was doing. Her parents agreed that the best thing to do was to talk to Craig's parents and get them to explain to Craig that having sex with Georgia was not appropriate. Her father assured her it wouldn't happen again.

Georgia's understanding was that when Craig's parents were approached, they dismissed the information by claiming that Craig was a very good boy and would never do such a thing; an answer that her parents seemed to accept. Craig was furious and made Georgia pay. She never told again.

Not only was the parental response woefully inadequate, the inadequacy continued in that nothing about the "Craig incident" was ever mentioned again.

Georgia's response to this parental failure was to go into herself and retreat. At about this time she became aware that she was hearing things that didn't seem "real." There was a voice in her head telling her to do bad things and telling her she was despicable. She also began seeing things, like giant spider webs in her garden that were peculiar.

Not surprisingly, she became increasingly withdrawn. Realising that she was totally on her own, she tried to kill herself by running into a busy road. She was struck by a car, but survived with a broken foot and significant soft tissue injuries.

Much to Georgia's later shame, this desperate suicide attempt was done in full view of her mother. This time, the parental response was quick and determined. Georgia was escorted to a psychiatrist.

Here Georgia reported that she was told what was wrong with her. She had a schizo-affective disorder and needed urgent hospitalisation. He pointed to her weird beliefs about her computer being hacked, the fact that she had command hallucinations and a voice that told her she was despicable. Georgia recalled that she was also told off: "Didn't she realise that she was really upsetting her parents?"

Although a minor, she was prescribed an anti-psychotic and a "mood stabilizer," Lamotrigine, that of course is not really a mood stabiliser at all, but rather a drug that is used in the management of epilepsy. Georgia found that her brain seized up.

Throughout numerous psychiatric consultations and admissions, no one, in any way, ever asked her, "What Happened To You?"

Mind you that was some fifteen years ago.

Yet, as Prof. Richard Bentall has recently written, it is surprising that psychiatric teams are only focusing on treating patients with medication, despite the fact that we know that environment and specific experiences are directly linked to the symptoms. He goes on to say that it is vital that psychiatric services question patients about their life experience.

Needless to say her hospitalisation did not result in any significant amelioration of her psychosis, largely because, as Georgia later told, she was terrified to go home because Craig was out there waiting. And wait he did. And rape her again he did.

In order to avoid him she started to run away from home and lived on the streets. This involved Georgia getting into a fight for survival that included shoplifting, riding on trains to pass the time and trading sex for shelter and food. By fifteen Georgia had learned that if you promise males sex but delay, you can nearly always get what you need. Georgia noted that every now and then she would be apprehended by the police and taken home, only to be pursued by Craig and later run away again. Georgia said she was surprised that no one ever asked why she ran away from home. It was deemed to be due to her schizo-affective mental illness.

While on the streets she often still attended school, enjoying the safety of her classroom. However, following a tense meeting with her parents and the principal, she was expelled because if she was not living at home, she was not welcome in the school. Her life became even more chaotic.

Not surprisingly, Georgia countered the increasingly nasty voices in her head by drinking and using methamphetamine. In amongst this chaos her occasional returns home often involved being Craig's unwillingly sexual partner. At sixteen she became pregnant to him.

She asked if she could come home, but this request was totally rejected by her father. Only special pleading by her mother allowed her to not be both pregnant and homeless.

Georgia said that being pregnant immediately sobered her up. Georgia informed her parents that the pregnancy was the outcome of partying with an unknown American sailor who was temporarily in port. She did however find the courage to ignore/resist Craig's attentions.

Following the pregnancy Georgia saw Craig only once more. She said she had taken the baby out for a walk only to realise Craig was watching her. She said she held her baby tight and hid behind a tree. He watched them for a while and then drove off.

Over the past decade Georgia has had multiple psychiatric admissions for her "schizo-affective disorder," for her "bipolar disorder" and her alcohol dependence. At one stage she was being prescribed four anti-psychotics, two mood stabilisers and an anti-depressant.

It is worth commenting on the use of so-called "anti-psychotics." Anti-psychotics are not "anti-psychotics." The first so-called "anti-psychotic" (Chlorpromazine) was discovered by chance in 1950 when being used by a surgeon as an anaesthetic. He noted that people on whom it was used became indifferent to their surroundings. Thus, it was gradually deemed suitable for use as an anti-agitation drug. It was also gradually found to be good for controlling vomiting and nausea, so in Europe it was called Largactil (for large action). It was subsequently realised that regular use of the drug appeared to not only quell agitation, but also dampened down psychotic symptoms, such as hallucinations. It is important to note that the two psychiatrists responsible for promulgating the use of Chlorpromazine did not view the drug as being an "anti-psychotic" or an even an anti-schizophrenic medication. Indeed, they correctly called chlorpromazine a "neuroleptic" or "brain seizing" drug. It is important to recognise that the plethora of drugs now called "anti-psychotics" do not cure or remove hallucinations. What they do is seize up the user's brains to such extent that they literally become indifferent to the still ongoing hallucinations. Although this brain seizing effect may be useful, the dampening effect is also accompanied by a nasty raft of effects, caused by the very action of neuroleptic drugs. All anti-psychotics reduce dopamine activity in the brain. As a consequence of this action the following can happen (from Healy 2016).

The list is long and horrible and includes:

- Stiffness/lack of movement (from clumsiness to zombie state)
- Abnormal movements, known as dyskinesias that mimic Parkinson's
- Abnormal muscle tone, known as dystonia where muscles go into spasm
- Restless, agitation or internal turmoil, known as akathisia
- Demotivation; a state of indifference
- Hormonal changes, mainly increased lactation in women or breast development in men
- Weight gain - this can be very significant, some patients increase their weight by ten to twenty percent
- Metabolic syndromes increase blood sugar lipid levels, may cause diabetes and subsequent cardiovascular complications
- Lowered blood pressure and sedation
- Dry mouth, blurring of vision
- Sexual dysfunction, loss of libido, delayed ejaculation, impotence
- Skin rashes
- Neuroleptic syndrome, becoming feverish, stiff, disorganised, dead
- Catatonia
- Cardiovascular impairments
- Epilepsy
- Suicide
- Severe withdrawal effects
- Bed wetting
- Tooth loss

Given the above it is not surprising that in a review of these "brain seizing" drugs Gotzsche (2017) wrote "anti-psychotics are some of the most toxic drugs ever invented." And Dr. Peter Breggin (2017) concurred, "the neuroleptic drugs are among the most toxic and deadly medicines in use today."

If all of the above was not problematic enough, one very common impact (forty to sixty percent of users) of the long-term use of "anti-psychotics" is tardive dyskinesia. Unlike the side-effects listed above, Tardive Dyskinesia can last for years after the cessation of the drug.

"Tardive Dyskinesia (TD) is a persistent usually irreversible neurological disorder caused by neuroleptic drugs. TD manifests in abnormal movements of any muscles that are wholly or partially under voluntary control including face, jaw, eyelids, tongue, neck, shoulders, back abdomen, extremities including hands and feet fingers and toes."

Furthermore, just like the so-called anti-depressants, there is now considerable evidence that the clinical benefits of using anti-psychotics have been highly over stated. Two major markers of this over statement are that there is no evidence to support the pervasive belief that the early treatment of first episode psychosis with anti-psychotics improves the outcome. A Cochrane review of this practice concluded, "The available evidence does not support the conclusion that anti-psychotic treatment, in an acute early episode of psychosis, is effective."

What is even more damning, is that in a study of the maintenance use versus reduction/cessation of "anti-psychotics," more people in the dose reduction/cessation group improved (forty percent) than that of the maintenance group (eighteen percent).

Richard Bentall (2010) wrote that is seems hard to justify the faith modern psychiatric services have in anti-psychotics, taking into account the very severe side effects.

Or, more succinctly, "My take on the thousands of trials that have been performed on the use of anti-psychotics is that we don't have the evidence to support using anti-psychotics at all." (Peter Gotzsche 2017).

The imbalance of the psychiatric profession's acceptance, belief in, and use of anti-psychotic drugs - writing as recently as 2015, Jeffrey Lieberman of *Shrinks* fame wrote about "the mindboggling effectiveness of psychiatric drugs," (that truly is mindboggling) - spills over into their day to day practice distorting the landscape of truth.

I was witness to Georgia's psychiatrist telling her with authority, clarity and total conviction that "the more psychotic episodes you have, the more you will damage your brain."

I was surprised by this, I did not know that psychosis caused brain damage, so I went and explored the evidence. Well, the psychiatrist was a bit right. The evidence is that "anti-psychotics" cause brain damage in a dose related manner. The more you use, and the greater the amounts you take, the more brain damaged you become.

Owing to Georgia's history and at times her somewhat precarious mental state in therapy, I focused on offering her a place of safety. Somewhere that she could just be.

Our therapy sessions were also a place of:

- Acceptance - "You were not 'dreadfully promiscuous,' but rather doing what you needed to in order to survive."
- Curiosity – "Tell me what happened?"
- Understanding - "Everyone who is placed under long term constant stress develops significant mental health issues."
- Empathy - "It must have been shockingly hard being you. I'm amazed you're alive."
- Love - "I really admire your bravery."
- … and Playfulness - "Oh, don't tell me you've been letting that perfect family of yours down again?"

We were also successful in nudging her parents into doing some family therapy. Albeit with a different therapist as I was not sure I would have been able to contain my counter transference distaste of them!

Georgia and I worked together in group and then individually for just over a two-year period, at which time, because of my retirement, I transitioned Georgia into working with an excellent colleague.

In writing this chapter, I asked to catch up with her and see how she was going.

We met for coffee. She is now thirty-one and lives with her teenage daughter, aided and abetted by her mother.

She is not psychotic. She takes no anti-psychotic medication.

Her only "psych meds" are 100mgs of Pristiq, an anti-depressant that she has taken for years and is contemplating coming off. Her mood varies and sometimes the appalling nature of her childhood catches up with her and she wants to die. However, she recalls that she cannot do that because if she does she will substantially increase the suicide risk of her daughter.

No longer being on anti-psychotics or Avanza, she has lost thirty kilos. Her bright, funny, engaging style hides a lot of shame and pain, but here is an attractive young woman that, unless you asked, you would never know "What Happened To Her."

My view is that Georgia is now ready to attempt some bodywork therapy and maybe try some Comprehensive Resource Model therapy. She is, I believe, thinking about it.

Funnily enough history does, some forty years on, repeat itself. As our coffee catch up concluded I asked her, "What was it about our therapy that worked for you?"

Without hesitation she replied, "I thought you liked me."

And I did, and I do.

Chapter Nine

"I want to die."

Freda was a perfect, unfortunate example of childhood neglect and abuse. Freda turned up to one of my outpatient groups. For some ten years, every Thursday, I ran a group called "Strive & Thrive." Or, S & T, for short, so-called because I was only too aware that if you have a very poor childhood, then you will in all probability have an adult life of striving but not, necessarily, thriving. This group was dedicated to helping adults with developmental trauma make as much repair as was humanly possible.

S & T was a psychotherapeutic, as opposed to a psycho-educational, group. In a psychotherapeutic group, the members set the agenda and do the work. In psycho-educational groups, the leader sets the agenda and guides the clients on the work that needs to be done.

I started every S & T group the same way. I would invite a member of the group to start the ball rolling. I'd have them introduce themselves, give a one sentence observation as to how they were travelling and make a statement. "My agenda for group today is …"

The ideal group number is seven plus or minus two. The attendance at S & T varied, but usually was around eight to ten. There was, therefore, a need to pace the group well so that all participants were involved.

Every week the composition of the group was different. There were always one or two new people and one or two of the regulars would be elsewhere. Additionally, over time some old hands would drop out of the group having decided that they had done enough (or had enough) group work.

Freda was, I found out later, in her late forties, but she looked older. She was obese. It quickly became apparent she was hard of hearing and lip read a lot. Her dress sense was non-descript.

When it came to Freda's turn to speak, she said her name and then in a low, sad voice said, "I want to die." Her agenda for the day was, "how to kill myself. I've tried lots of times. I haven't got it right yet."

Every therapist has counter transference issues. As Freda uttered the words, "I want to die," my teeth clenched. Her agenda on successful suicide infuriated me. I wanted to slap her and say, "I can tell you how. The railway line is 250 metres from here."

My father was a police officer. He tolerated no nonsense, especially not from his children. Being pathetic was not allowed. You got on with things. You made do. You covered up your feelings. You were never vulnerable. You didn't show weakness. You made the best of things. Such a psychological perspective worked well for him; but then he had been brought up in an orphanage.

My visceral response to Freda was familiar. Every now and then, my "you're being pathetic" button would be triggered. The trick of being able to catch (bracket your own emotional reactions) is crucial. I instantly knew I would need to be on my absolute best game with Freda.

I also knew right then and there that I was going to go out of my way to save her life. I would haul her back from the brink of extinction. I was hooked. I knew what it was like to be deemed pathetic.

I had three older sisters who nicknamed me after one of the characters in the BBC Children's television show *Bill and Ben the Flower Pot Men*. That character was "Little Weed." I still recall walking into my big sister's house in Northampton one night some forty years later as a big grown up and being greeted with the epithet "Hello Little Weeeeeeed."

I said, "Freda, Welcome to S & T. I am saddened to hear how distressed you are. I hope that the group today will offer you some solace."

I invited the rest of the group members to say their piece. After everyone had spoken my usual practice was to remember and recap the presented agendas. It was often possible to find from the stated agendas psychological commonalities, or at least common running threads. I would then throw whatever seemed to be the most consensual agenda up in the air for discussion.

However, not this day. When the last patient had spoken, I said, "Who in this room has ever wanted to die?"

As it happened that day we had two trainee postgraduate psychology students "sitting in" on the group. Everyone put a hand up.

"See Freda, you are not alone. Let's talk about wanting to die."

The following hour was an intense, emotional and invigorating one. A very useful trick in working with people is to remember that the most soothing antidote to distress is to talk. Many dependent drug users would, of course, deny this. They know that heroin, or alcohol or cannabis are much more effective. Well, they certainly work quicker than talking, but talking about distress is what emotionally regulated people do and it is the optimum antidote. A group is the ideal place to practice talking.

As the group explored the wish to die, a key theme emerged - yes, at times you may want to die, may really want to die, but such feelings pass.

One of the post grad students talked of her own suicide attempt (a stiff overdose of tricyclic "anti-depressant" pills) and of her disappointment at coming round in an ICU. However, in recovery, when it became possible that the very drugs she had used to overdose may have sufficiently damaged her liver so that over the next month or so she could die, she reported that she became totally terrified at the prospect.

As the time for a coffee break neared, I asked Freda about her experience of being in group that morning. The phrase is very useful. If you ask a patient "How was group today?" You inevitably get a logical, "good," "a bit boring," "great," or "interesting." But, if you ask: "What was your *experience* of being in group today?" You get a very different quality of response.

Freda said, "I'm glad I came. I didn't want to. It's good not to be on my own with this."

After the break the group continued with the theme of suicide and the impact that suicide had on others. There was a strong discussion on whether suicide was a selfish act. Freda said it would be a relief. This gave me an opening to ask my favourite suicide question. "Freda," I said, "at this moment, how much of you wants to die? Give the group a percentage."

She paused and thought.

She countered, "You mean right now?"

"Yes, right now."

"Seventy percent," she said.

I continued. "How about when you came into the group this morning?"

"Ninety-five percent," she said.

The previously suicidal postgrad student said, "Um, yes that's the problem isn't it? Your 'wanting to die index' changes." (She was after all a psychologist). "You can't rely on the fact that the next day you won't feel different."

I corrected her. "Actually you can, it changes all the time. That's why you can never be sure killing yourself is the right decision."

I then deployed a favourite trick of the trade. I said to Freda, "When you say that ninety five percent of you wants to die, or that seventy-five percent of you wants to die, what is that other left over, however small, percentage saying to you?"

She paused, she shook her head and slowly said, "It says not yet, things might improve, this is not the end, there is hope."

In his entertaining and insightful book, *This Is How*, Augusten Burroughs describes one of his own suicide attempts. He wrote that aged fourteen he had decided to kill himself because it would bring him relief. He placed both of his wrists under a hot tap and scalded them until they were numb. However, as he prepared to slit his now numb wrists with a razor blade, he realised that rather than end peacefully, his last moments would be of total panic and misery as his reptilian brain watched the blood pouring from his slit wrists. Burroughs wrote cleverly, "It wasn't that I wanted to kill myself, it was that I wanted to end my life."

The next day Augusten Burroughs ended his current life not by death, but by the decision to walk out of his house, change his name to Augusten and become an author. "I hate my life" is not the same as "I want to die."

So I borrowed from the good Augusten and said to Freda, "How much do you hate your life?"

She looked startled, then wept. "I hate it totally. It's appalling."

Again, as Augusten Burroughs has aptly noted, "The dishonesty that resides inside suicide is that there are no other options."

My experience is that what changes your "wanting to die index" is connection. Connection to people, connection to someone who will listen; attachment is the answer. Sometimes, the only person able to provide connection is a therapist. Sometimes you are all they have. That is the honour and the burden of being a therapist.

The best option for suicidal thinking is definitely not a pill. "Anti-depressants" have a well documented risk of increasing suicidality. Indeed, in any randomised controlled trial of "anti-depressants," there are always more dead bodies in the group given the "anti-depressant" than in the control placebo group given, for example, Vitamin C or a sugar pill.

Given that people who have had adverse childhood experiences have a hugely increased risk of suicide, it is necessary for any therapist working with traumatised people to have a clear policy on suicide.

Mine is that I will do all I can to stop it. I will intervene. I will pull all the levers to obstruct people from dying.

I can understand that if someone is in terminal physical pain, then a doctor-assisted death is desirable. I too will also book my flight to Switzerland. However, I will not allow emotional pain, emotional distress, emotional dysregulation that is the cause of suicidal thoughts or action to be perceived as the same as a terminal illness.

The reason is that being very distressed, being very unhappy, hating one's life is not an illness. It is a consequence of your childhood, a consequence that can be ameliorated. Psychotherapy works. It is the most effective intervention for emotional pain. Emotional pain can be managed, can be lessened, and can be removed.

Additionally, I have never had a patient whose suicide attempt, if thwarted, has not, some months later, been pleased that they are still alive.

I said to Freda, "Please watch this."

I then asked the group, "If you have attempted suicide in the past please raise your hand."

Eight out of the group of twelve did so (including both of the psych students and Freda).

"Now lower your hands if you are pleased that your suicide attempt was *not* successful."

Everyone but Freda lowered their hands.

There is a dogma that has, unfortunately, become an absolute truth. It is taught in Psychology and I suspect other counselling courses. This absolute truth is:

NEVER GIVE YOUR PHONE NUMBER TO A PATIENT.

I can understand that twenty years ago or so, before the universal use of mobile phones, that such advice was sound. When you only had a home landline then not revealing that was wise. But now that we all have mobile phones I think the rule needs revision.

I always give my patients my mobile number. It is on my business card.

I boundary it by saying that I am a 7am to 7pm service. (Though of late that's crept to being an 8am to 7pm service, then to an 8am to 5pm service: getting old has an impact.)

I am also clear that if a patient is having suicidal thoughts then we can explore that in the next session.

However, I say, "If you are seriously thinking of trying to kill yourself, if the idea is becoming very appealing, then take yourself to your nearest ED. But, if you are *dying*, then call me."

Here are four, totally true examples, of why giving patients a mobile phone number is a legitimate ethical and necessary aspect of the business of being a therapist working with traumatised adults.

I was out to dinner with a colleague. My phone rang. If I have clients about whom I have concerns about suicide I add their mobile numbers to my phone. Just in case. On this occasion I can see it is a client with a past history of suicide.

"Hi Jackson, how you going?"

"I can't go on Bill, I've had a row with dad and then Susan," (Jackson's partner), "So that's it. Thanks for all your help. Goodbye Bill."

On my phone I have an app that allows me access to my electronic patient database. I looked him up. I called the Police. I call their call centre not the emergency line. 000 or 999 are less useful than being able to talk to a police operator directly.

WHAT HAPPENED?

I informed them that a Jackson Coates of such and such address, and date of birth, had just called me and made a serious suicide threat. I also informed them that in all probability he was intoxicated and could be down by the river near to his home address. I was aware from my sessions with him that when distressed, he often took himself off to the river. I warned them that he was a butcher and that he may have sharp knives to hand. I warned them that he had in the past spoken of a "shot by cop" suicide.

I went back to dinner. Some two hours or so later, as my colleague and I were leaving the restaurant, my phone rang. I answered. The caller identified himself as a police sergeant and said that the patient was now being taken to an Emergency Department. Unfortunately, I didn't pay much attention to the name of the sergeant.

A few days later Jackson's dad called the office and made an appointment for his son to see me. When I saw Jackson I said, "How's your world?"

He smiled ruefully. "Well, I'm still here."

"Would you like to tell me what happened?"

Jackson said that he was in dark despair. Following his altercation with his dad, his pregnant partner had, he felt, taken dad's side. He felt betrayed and very angry. He had parked down by the river and was sitting in the back of his ute having a few beers. He said he had his knives with him and was waiting for the alcohol to kick in, then he was going to wade into the river, slice his wrists open and float away to die.

He was sitting in dark contemplation when a somewhat shabby bloke wearing a mac walked past the back of his ute. The stranger said, "Hey, good day mate."

Jackson, taken a bit by surprise, said, "Oh, hi."

The stranger said, "You wouldn't have a spare beer would you?"

Jackson said he wanted to tell the stranger to "fuck off," but his good manners prevented him. (He had a very strict, hard-working father).

"Yes, sure," he said.

The stranger climbed on board. They chatted a bit and drank a beer. The stranger thanked him for the beer and then said to him, "Oh, you have some very cool knives there."

Jackson reported that he'd said something like, "Yes, I'm a butcher. They are good, aren't they?"

The stranger then said, "Mate, you're not thinking of killing yourself, are you?"

Jackson, taken by complete surprise, said, "Well, yes."

The stranger said, "I know mate. I've been there. I felt like that a year or so ago. My wife left me, the job you know, said I was never home. It was a very tough year. But, I'm okay now."

Jackson said, "Oh, that's shit, what's your job?"

The stranger said, "I'm a police officer, and I'm here to take you to hospital."

I wish I paid more attention to his name. Jackson is alive today.

The second was less dramatic, but nonetheless life-saving. I was five minutes away from home one evening. My phone rang. It was one minute to seven.

"Hi, Sheila," I said. Her reply was a slurry of words but I heard, "Bill, I'm dying."

"Where are you?"

"In a park, in my car, goodbye."

She hung up.

I rang back. She answered.

I sternly asked, "Which park?"

My question, maybe the authority in my tone, I think unsettled her.

"Oh," she said, "King's Park."

I hung up. The police found her unconscious thirty minutes later.

She is alive today.

And now for the absolutely most spectacular, you just wouldn't believe it, totally true, incident.

I was out to dinner with a colleague. It was ten to seven. My phone rang.

"Hi Rosie," I said.

"He's a fucker bill, he's a total fucker, that's it, I'm done."

I could hear from her breathing that she was exerting herself.

I said, "Oh Rosie, I'm sorry, where are you?"

"You know the place, I told you. That's it, I'm gone."

With that I heard her gasp and there was a crunch of noises. I assumed she had dropped her phone.

I instantly ended her call and called the police. I told them my name and informed the police operator that a Ms Rosie Alexander was in a very agitated, distressed state and was, in all probability, walking up from her house to an adjacent disused quarry from where she was intending to jump and kill herself. The police operator put me on hold, but in less than thirty seconds was back.

"Dr. Saunders, can you please speak to Sergeant Reynolds?"

"Eh, yes, of course." I waited, somewhat surprised at this unusual turn of events. A moment or two passed as we were connected.

Sergeant Reynolds said, "Dr. Saunders we have Rosie with us, she's safe and sound. We were just passing by and saw her fall into a drainage ditch, so we stopped to see if she was okay. Do you want to speak to her?"

"Yes, of course."

Rosie came on the line. She was furious.

"How the fuck did you do that? What are you? Fucking magic or what?"

I couldn't resist it. "Well Rosie, when it comes to you, of course, I'm fucking magic!"

Rosie was taken by the police to the nearest ED. She was admitted and some three days later released. She is alive (and still kicking) today.

Finally, in this justification of why patients get my phone, here is case number four.

I had a patient, Derek, who was a traumatised, retired police officer. He had, about a decade earlier, responded to an urgent domestic violence call and as he and his partner approached the house, a very angry man with a rifle ran from the side of the house and shot Derek's partner. Derek was for the next five hours held hostage at gunpoint by a very disorganised, psychotic man. Derek spent those five hours knowing that at any moment he could be shot.

He never returned to active policing. As he said, "I may not have been shot, but my nerves were."

Following his medical retirement from the police, Derek found it difficult to work. He was hypervigilant, depressed, anxious and had flashbacks, nightmares and intrusive thoughts about that day. He was a classic case of Post Traumatic Stress Disorder (PTSD).

We worked hard on Derek's trauma, but the use of EMDR, the optimum intervention for "one-off" life threatening trauma, was only partially useful. Unfortunately, Derek had had a very scary childhood (angry, ex-military father), so the hostage trauma sat on top of a raft of early childhood experiences of physical abuse.

Derek's overwhelming distress related to him being useless and not being able to provide for two teenage daughters. He was divorced and his ex-wife had her own issues with alcohol and benzodiazepine dependence. Derek told me he had a reasonable life insurance policy, but suicide was listed as an exclusion.

A further complication was that Derek had a chronic and unusual respiratory complaint. He managed this by the daily use of steroids. So, he hit on a plan. He decided to stop taking his steroids in the expectation that in a period of some three to four weeks the fluid in his lungs would build up and he would die from respiratory failure.

A great plan, apart from the fact that we have three brains. Logically, Derek wanted to die, so the insurance money would go to his kids. Emotionally, Derek felt so miserable about his existence that he wanted to die to gain relief from his self-loathing and his sense of appalling ineptitude.

However, we also have a reptilian brain. After some five to six weeks of not using his steroid medication, Derek woke up gasping for breath.

Although he had been aware over the previous week or so that his breathing was becoming compromised, he had taken satisfaction in the knowledge that his plan was working. However, this was now very different. Every breath required huge effort. His reptilian brain kicked in. Suddenly, dying was terrifying. In a total panic he phoned me. Of course an ambulance would have been a much better idea, but panic is not logical.

I took his call on the way to work. He begged for help. I asked him for his address. Amazingly I realised that I was literally a street away. When I arrived he was gasping for breath. He was turning blue. Too late, I thought, for that ambulance. The nearest ED was about ten minutes away. I bundled him into my car. I phoned a medical colleague and asked if there was anything I should be doing. He said, "Drive faster." I did. My colleague alerted the nearest ED. On arrival there were two paramedics with a gurney waiting for us. He was whisked away.

I love it when the world works properly.

The respiratory doctor later told Derek that his survival had been touch and go.

Derek is still alive today. I know that because about two years ago when walking through a local university on my way to teach medical students I saw him. I waved. He smiled. He said he was on his way to hand in his last assignment for his law degree.

However, you don't always get it right.

One evening when at work running a men's group, I noticed in the break that I had a text from Natalie, a patient with a very unpleasant childhood. Her father (British, ex-military) had made her life a misery. She reported that his favourite words to her as a child were, "You're pretty. Pretty dumb, pretty ugly, pretty stupid." She had, perhaps needless to say, married a man who also abused her. Now separated, she was struggling financially and emotionally. Her text to me read:

"I know I have to do it. I'm scared, but I will do it. Thank you."

I read this just as I was about to re-enter group. I did not have time to phone her, so I phoned the police and asked them to undertake a welfare check. Which, they did. Later, as I was writing up my group notes, I got a phone call from Natalie. She was in an ED. She said to me, "You forgot didn't you?"

"Sorry, forgot what Nat?"

"That tomorrow I'm having my knee replaced. I was texting you about the operation!"

Fortunately, after an assessment, she was allowed to go home.

Interestingly, when we later caught up and I apologised for my mistake, she said, "No worries, thank you for caring about me."

Suicide prevention has become a buzz word, but suicide rates are increasing. Perhaps as therapists we just need to be a bit braver, a bit less protocol-ed. So, if you work as a therapist, give people your mobile phone number. Of course, put in some boundaries. Of course, guide patients on how to use it, not abuse it.

Having written the above, I went and checked my electronic case notes. I reviewed the names of all the people I had seen over the previous seven years. I counted ten patients (including the above) who I could remember intervening in their lives and preventing their deaths. Of the ten, eight are still alive. Just imagine if every therapist of whatever persuasion adopted the above practice, then that really would constitute suicide prevention.

Chapter Ten

The man who wanted to kill and eat me

I opened the referral letter and burst out laughing. The referral from a psychiatric colleague was blunt and to the point.

Dear Bill,
Re Mr. John Smith, (21/3/1975)
Please see the above. He is a cannibal.
Yours sincerely,
David.

I showed the letter to our hard-working, always keen to get things right, practice manager. "See," I said, "everyone makes mistakes. This guy is obviously cannabis dependent. The secretary has clearly made a typo! Please give Mr. Smith the next available appointment."

Some three weeks later, Mr. Smith was my two o'clock patient. Exactly on time, I left my office and stepped into the waiting room. There was one male patient sitting waiting. I approached him and said, "I'm Bill Saunders, come on in."

It is important to be on time, every time. This is the patient's hour (well, fifty minutes) and punctuality conveys that you take them seriously. Time management is all about priority, and it's important to convey to the patient that they are the priority.

I allowed Mr. Smith to enter my room first. I always do that. You can learn heaps about a patient by how they address the issue of where to sit.

Mr. Smith duly raised his eyebrows and said, "Shall I sit on the sofa?"

WHAT HAPPENED?

I have a big, very comfortable, three seater sofa. Sometimes patients will sprawl, some sit neatly, some will be just on the edge, some sit back and relax. It's all good information. I smiled and gesturing toward the sofa said, "Yes, please take a seat."

On occasions, a new patient will just walk into the room and, without questioning, just sit down. On a few occasions, some have opted for my chair. I make no comment and sit on the sofa. But, just as those that ask the question, the seat stealers have conveyed to me an aspect of their nature.

I use the same room for all my sessions; and the room is always the same. I keep everything in the same place. Even the books in the bookcase are put back exactly where they were pulled from. The room is tidy. The pictures on the wall are abstracts. This may sound finicky, but it's important. Bringing patients into exactly the same room every time gives them a sense of safety. There are no surprises. This is especially important when working with adults who have been severely traumatised in childhood.

One day, when browsing around a bookshop I discovered that they sold knick knacks including cushions. I found two brightly coloured flower design cushions. I instantly liked them. I thought, "Ha, this will brighten up my room." I duly put them on each end of the sofa. They were very fetching.

The first patient after the installation of the cushions commented, "Hey, great cushions." The second made no comment at all and the third, a woman who had been repeatedly sexually abused by her father, screamed. It became a matter of honour between us that on every one of her visits, I would remove the cushions before she entered the room.

There is another issue about being a therapist. That is what you wear. Over the years I developed a therapy uniform. I wear black trousers, a blue striped shirt, black socks, black shoes and a ring on the fourth finger of both hands. Plus my all-important glasses and then, more recently, discreet hearing aids.

My reason for so doing is if I am the same for every patient (and the room is the same for every patient), then I have a consistent backdrop against which to assess every patient. If a repeat patient is different in presentation, then it is not me, or the room that has influenced them. Similarly, if a new patient comes in, anything they say about me or the room is excellent information about them.

I recall one patient who exclaimed on meeting me for the first time, "Oh, you are darker than I thought you would be." He never came for a second appointment.

So I said to Mr. Smith, "Welcome, what brings you to see a psychologist?"

He calmly replied, "I want to kill and eat someone."

Although somewhere in the back of my brain I thought, "Oh fuck, he *is* a cannibal," a very important trick of psychotherapy is to accept everything that is presented to you as though it is perfectly normal. Thus, being a potential cannibal is an unremarkable everyday event.

There is a need to keep an inscrutable, impervious façade. Leak nothing, but curiosity, interest, acceptance and empathy for the client's dilemma. It is absolutely essential that you not recoil with disgust or in any way leak your disapproval.

My absolutely most surprising and shocking opening response from a client occurred when a new patient (Jane) in response to my "What brings you to see a psychologist?" said, "I've been depressed for fifteen years."

Now, from having asked that question hundreds of times, I knew straight away that her response was very unusual so I went straight to where she had pointed. "Jane, what happened fifteen years ago?"

She looked at the ground and quietly said, "I came home early from work and my husband was having sex with our German Shepard."

"What did you do?"

"We got the dog put down."

"How's your relationship with your husband now?"

She paused, "Ah, it's sort of okay."

Longer pause, and then a vacant, "We have two male poodles now."

Although I was stunned by her responses, I did my best to remain as though nothing shocking had been said and that what had occurred was entirely reasonable.

If one is feeling judgemental, censorious, offended, confronted, or disgusted about what a patient has said, a trick of the trade is to deploy curiosity. Deploy lots of it. Become totally invested in understanding. The capacity to suspend judgement, indeed, to become fascinated by that which offends your personal susceptibilities, is a hallmark feature of being able to establish and maintain a therapeutic relationship.

I became totally intrigued. I sat and explored with her. If you place yourself in the role of a mind detective, suspend your judgement and explore, everything will eventually become understandable. The best work, the best moments in therapy, are when you and patient sit together and work out why he or she is as they are.

Of course, the patient knew she had done the wrong thing. She hated herself even more for being so weak as to stay with her husband. Her self-loathing was literally tangible. However, the question, of course, was not to blame herself but to understand herself.

I have a catch phrase, "gently, gently" that I kindly chastise patients with when they lurch into self-blame or self-hatred. I used it a lot with Jane.

Self-compassion is the true antidote to self-loathing. I have in my desk a sheaf

WHAT HAPPENED?

of A4 pages. Each one has written in big type:
NEVER, NEVER, NEVER, EVER,
(Don't even think about it)
NEVER, EVER, CRITICISE YOURSELF.

I think I must have handed Jane a hundred of them. The first time she silently read it and tore it up. "That's stupid," she said. By the last time she laughed and said, "I know, I'll take it home and add it to the pile of others."

Jane slowly and hesitantly told her story. Her husband had literally rescued her at sixteen from a sexually abusive father and a totally insipid, passive, mother. They met when she was waiting in a fish and chip shop for the family dinner. He was also waiting. Fifteen years older than her, he had remarked, "Hey, why so sad?" She reported that she had looked up, startled, and burst in to tears.

As he left the shop with his fish and chips, he handed her his business card and said, "If you ever want to talk, call me. I hate seeing a beautiful girl cry."

She reported that she was nonplussed, bewildered; her a beautiful girl? Impossible.

She telephoned him a day later. A month later she left her family home forever. She never saw her parents again. She moved in with him. Unfortunately, many traumatised patients leap out of the frying pan of one abusive relationship into the fire of another.

Over the course of therapy she slowly accepted that standing up for herself and doing what was good for her was very hard. Indeed, her childhood had been one in which giving into the needs of her sexually predatory father was the safe option. Resistance was futile. At age ten when she told her mum about dad's sexual abuse, mum told her to stop telling stories. If she resisted dad he became violent. The safe thing was to go along with the abuse.

One thing you quickly learn as a therapist is that the defences people use as a child to keep themselves psychologically and physically safe become, as an adult, hurtful and harmful.

Jane was a classic exemplar of this. As a child doing what the other wanted kept her safe. As an adult, doing what her husband wanted drove her literally crazy.

Slowly Jane started to put boundaries in place. She hesitantly pushed back against the demands of her husband and their stay-at-home adult son. She learned that saying no was possible. Especially if you do it when you first want to, and not weeks later when saying no is always so much harder, and always brings so much resistance.

She applied for, and got, a more senior administrative job at the university where she worked. She entered and ran a twelve kilometre city to surf race and proudly reported she hadn't come last. Finally, at the age of sixty, she walked out of the marital house and never went back.

This time no one had to rescue her. She did it herself. In our last appointment she said, "Hey, I had a really strange feeling the other day. I was sitting on the beach watching my grandchild play. This weird feeling came over me. It made my heart race. I think I was happy."

So, Mr. Smith's revelation that he wanted to kill and eat people engendered in me intrigue. I deployed my impervious, this-is-an-everyday-matter façade and said, "You want to do that because?"

Mr. Smith responded, "Because I've eaten just about every other animal on the planet so eating a human would complete the list."

Ah well, if you don't at first succeed …

"And you want to complete the list, because?"

"Because I think I can."

"And would be important for you because?"

Mr. Smith looked at me intently, "Because I think I could get away with it."

I was tempted to ask another because, but my experience with "becauses" is that three is the limit.

So I changed tack, a little, but used what he had given me.

"So, you're telling me that getting away with things appeals to you."

He nodded.

I deployed, what I hoped was a "gotcha," question.

"So," I paused slightly, "as a kid, was it really difficult to get away with things?"

He paused, laughed and said, "Hey, did you know my dad?"

I love "gotcha" questions. The trick when asking questions in therapy is never to think of your next question. Listen to understand. Don't listen to be able to reply. Sit and be with the patient. Listen. And, lo and behold, something will just pop into your head. Sometimes my questions even surprise me. If nothing comes to mind, sit and wait. The patient will usually fill the space. When teaching students, I always tell them the first skill to learn was to "shut the fuck up and listen."

Given that I had a background from my apprenticeship in The Alcoholism Treatment Unit in Glasgow, I find that "gotcha" questions relating to patient's drug use are especially delightful.

One patient, an entertaining cardiologist with an imperious drinking problem (that he was very reluctant to own) told me after my "How's your world?" opening that "Things were good."

It transpired that he was four weeks sober, he was sleeping better, his relationship with his wife was more harmonious, he was exercising more, had lost weight and even his liver was improving.

I said, "Well, that's a bummer, isn't it?"

Surprised, he said, "What do you mean?"

WHAT HAPPENED?

I said, "It means that you do have a problem with alcohol."

"Bugger," he said.

So, getting back to Mr. Smith, I said, "Tell me about your dad."

Mr. Smith's dad was a coal miner. He was big, very hard-working and brutal. Raised in the North of England, Mr. Smith recalled that an hour before his father's arrival home from the pit, his mother would ensure that everything was in place. He and his two younger brothers were literally told to sit absolutely still and do nothing. In the meantime, his mother would attempt to make the house as tidy as possible while simultaneously cooking dinner. Mr. Smith noted that because he was the oldest, he was charged by his father to ensure that his two young brothers behaved.

Life was extremely regimented. His father demanded order. He recalled that Mondays were the days his mum did the washing. Tuesdays were ironing days. Wednesdays were housework days and Thursdays shopping days. Fridays were the worst. His father would be paid at the end of his shift and come home after "a couple of pints" in the pub. His father demanded respect. He was the person whose labour paid for everything. They needed to adhere to his rules. Saturdays were also fraught. His father was a die-hard Middlesbrough United Football supporter. The results dictated his father's mood and the well-being in the house.

Mr. Smith reported that his father had rules about everything. Any infractions, noise, fighting, disrespect, "giving lip," being late, breaking things, not answering properly or promptly, resulted in six swipes of the cane onto bare legs or buttocks. Mr. Smith said being caned became so normal, an almost daily occurrence, that he learned to endure it without complaint.

He noted without rancour, "You just have to go with the rhythm of the beatings."

I remember asking him my favourite "B & Q" question (or "Bunnings" when working in Australia).

"If you go to B & Q and you can't find something you need, what do you do?"

He immediately said, "I go up and down the aisles searching for it. I always find it in the end."

My experience is that people who have had abusive childhoods never ask for help. Indeed, why would they? No one helped them as a child. So learning to be totally self-reliant is protective. But that which keeps you safe as a child, becomes hurtful and harmful as an adult.

Mr. Smith noted that by the time he was ten he felt nothing. He was, he said, "immune to his life." He thought that his mum had done her best, but she never protected him or his brothers from, or protested about, the beatings. Sometimes, she would even *tell* his dad to beat them.

He noted with a sigh, "But then she got some good beatings too."

As he moved into his teenage years he realised that he was different to most of the people around him. He realised that people often got upset, got angry, felt sad. He said that there was an accident at the mine where his dad worked and four miners were killed. Apart from thinking "pity it wasn't dad," he was surprised by the outpouring of grief and distress that people showed. He noted that he didn't understand it.

By the time he was fifteen, he was six foot two inches tall, and strong. He played football at school, but found boxing particularly enjoyable. He noted that being punched didn't hurt. He realised he loved violence. He loved what his violence did; it gave him control. It gave him power. He became very good at it.

When he was sixteen, his dad went to beat him for coming in late for dinner. Mr. Smith reported, with no little satisfaction, that he knocked his dad out with one punch. He was never hit again.

As I worked with Mr. Smith I reflected with him on his lack of feelings. He said it was "an annoyance;" a lack of something that he knew others had. He reported that the family dog had been run over. He told me quite calmly that because the dog had a broken leg, he shot it and placed the body in the rubbish bin. He was amazed when his young son came home, burst into tears, and called him "heartless."

However, he countered such annoyance by noting that at times it worked for him. He told me a story about being in a pub with a mate, although he also acknowledged he really only had acquaintances. As he and his "mate" were drinking, a group of some six males on an adjacent table became increasingly boisterous. Their noise annoyed him. He said that he looked over and ascertained who was the ringleader. After a further explosion of noise, he stood up and walked up to the identified ringleader. He said, "You have a choice. You can leave the pub now, or you can die."

"What happened?" I asked.

"Oh, they left the pub, quick sharp. He knew I would have killed him."

Some weeks later I was camping. A group of young men camping nearby, decided to party. I was furious about the noise they were making. At two in the morning I could stand it no more. I got out of my tent to confront them. I was very angry. I saw that there were about eight of them. They were young and fit. Although angry, I knew any confrontation would result in me being hurt.

I wished Mr. Smith had been there. He'd have sorted it. As has been noted by British psychologist Kevin Dutton, "When the stakes are high and backs are against the wall, it's a psychopath you want alongside you."

Mr. Smith reported that his unemotional use of violence gave him immense power. He said, "It's funny you know. People get angry and all emotional and then want to fight. But for me I never get angry. For me violence is merely an instrument to get what I want."

He also reported that when he was nineteen he had joined the army. It was a way of escaping his family and finding another one where he fitted in better. He quickly succeeded. He became a sergeant in the SAS and was deployed to Iraq as a sniper. He calmly reported that the action plan in any contact with the enemy was always to shoot the second most senior officer in the head. "Just like a watermelon exploding." He said, "You then waited for a medic to turn up, and shot them in the stomach. As they writhed around screaming, all the others would just run away. Your team could then advance."

Mr. Smith said this was the most satisfactory part of his life. He married a girl he met on the Internet, because "she seemed to like me. That was nice." He had a son, but volunteered for other assignments and was often away from home. Unfortunately, while deployed in Afghanistan his unit came under attack and in the confusion he was literally run over by an armoured car. He sustained a fractured pelvis. After "months in hospital" he was invalided out of the army.

He noted that the army was where he felt at home. Suddenly, he was, he said, "a displaced person."

He said that he missed the adrenalin of stalking the enemy, a sense of being alive; hunter or hunted. He could, in the army, absolutely get away with murder. On his discharge he went big game hunting. He got to eat some of his kills. He wondered whether stalking and eating a human would bring him back to life.

Over time, we had formed a connection in our sessions. He reported that he had never talked to anyone like he did with me.

Then, in what turned out to be our last session, he asked me to write in my notes that he was going to kill and eat me. I knew he meant it.

I asked why I needed to do that.

"Because," he said in a tone that conveyed it was obvious, "then I won't kill and eat you! You are not worth going to jail for!"

I looked at Mr. Smith.

"I'm not going to do that."

"Why not? It will save your life."

"Because I think you like me."

We sat quietly together.

The opposite of self-reliance is mutual inter-dependence.

At the end of the session I did something I almost never do. I stood up and gave him a hug. He stiffened. He left without a word.

He missed his next appointment. I asked the secretary to follow up and give him another. She couldn't contact him by phone. I sent him a letter inviting him to call my mobile number. Nothing happened. I stalked him; I drove out to his house. It looked empty.

I phoned the prison services to see if he had been incarcerated. He was not a prisoner. I checked the death notices. I Googled him. He had completely disappeared.

To this day, I wonder whether not doing as he requested was a mistake that made him terminate our contact. I wondered whether the intimacy we had established was too risky for him; hence, the threat to kill me.

I have also just fleetingly wondered if he had disappeared to save my life.

However, as my supervisor said when I discussed this case with him, "Come on Bill, he probably just got fed up seeing you and went and saw someone else!"

Though when talking about an adult male patient who has been abused in childhood, I think British psychiatrist Anthony Storr may have got it right when he said: "To accept love, is to place himself in a position of dependence so humiliating that he feels himself to be despicably weak."

Chapter Eleven

Pixie packs them in

Shame is the most toxic and corrosive of all emotions.
It cripples, it reduces, and annihilates its owner. Never mind Iago's warning to Othello to "beware of jealousy my lord, it mocks the meat it feeds upon," shame *eats* the meat it feeds upon. Be totally aware of your shame, because it will always gnaw away at you and stop you in your tracks.

Yet shame can be eliminated.

Sam came to group. A tall, lithe, fifty-year-old woman who, although physically attractive, was psychologically broken. Her eye contact was downcast, her demeanour shrivelled. She was difficult to engage and easy to ignore. Yet, she kept coming to my S & T group. After the sixth or so visit, I decided to take the bull by the proverbial horns.

"Sam," I said, "you are a bit of enigma. You have come to the last six or so groups yet although you are in plain sight you have remained invisible. Tell us about you."

It is always useful in a psychotherapeutic group to allow "hog sessions." That is one patient may, because of their current difficulties, "hog" a session and take up an hour or two of the group's time on their own issues.

Although, with this case, it was different. Here was a chameleon being "forced" into the visible glare of group scrutiny, yet the underlying theme was the same; you are valuable, you are worthwhile, we will all hear you.

My experience is also that reticence in group, that quiet withdrawal, is not about not wishing to speak, but being too ashamed to speak.

"What would you like to know?" said Sam.

I countered, "Whatever you would like to tell us."

Sam hesitated and said quietly, "I used to be a junkie, I used to be a prostitute and then I was a wife and now I don't know who I am."

I felt the group wait, as I was, for more.

Silence.

Sometimes you wait, sometimes you nudge. I waited, nothing, so then I nudged.

"Tell us about being a junkie."

Sam looked ahead and succinctly told the group that from the age of fourteen she had been a "pothead" and then, with access via her criminally inclined boyfriend, she had her first introduction to heroin.

"How was that?" I queried.

"Magnificent," she replied. "My boyfriend injected me, I was apprehensive, you hear bad things about smack, but it was marvellous. I knew it was in my body, I could sort of feel it and then it suddenly hit my brain and my brain just dissolved into an abyss of bliss. I'd never felt so secure, so whole, so calm, so wonderful. I was in a bubble, a cocoon, where nothing bad could get me. I said to my boyfriend this is amazing, I love it, it's wonderful, why didn't you tell me how good this shit is!"

I said, "Yes, that beautiful oblivion is magic isn't it?"

Sam nodded and said, "Yes, it's beautiful, but that's the trap, it was so beautiful, so wonderful, so enveloping, that it was evil."

It is always essential to see beyond the substance. Many people use opiates, only a minority become dependent.

"Sam, tell us why you think you found heroin so beguiling, so evil?"

For the first time Sam looked me straight in the eye and said, "Because just for the moment, it obliterated my shame."

Shame can lead to a shit load of problems.

Shame is one of those group topics that need to be handled carefully. It is the improvised explosive device of topics. If you don't take absolute precaution, it can blow up in your face.

I quickly scanned the group. Was this a safe place for Sam to share and explore her shame? I wasn't certain. There were two new members in group that day who, although on the surface looked agreeable, were unknown qualities, and then there was also Martha. Martha was a complex client whose history of childhood neglect and sexual abuse made her unpredictable, sometimes compassionate, sometimes rageful. Trauma breeds rage.

"Sam," I said, "thank you for letting us get to know a bit about you. I know telling what we don't like about ourselves can be challenging. What I am going to suggest is that next week we have a group that spends the whole day exploring shame."

The group positively acquiesced. Shame is an excellent topic for a psychotherapeutic group because the antidote, the vaccine for the venom of shame, is vulnerability and a big bright searchlight. However, the vaccine needs to be very carefully, very safely applied.

So I invited the new comers to tell something of themselves, and then the group explored what people needed to feel safe in next week's shame group. Trust, acceptance, curiosity, confidentiality, honesty, being non-judgemental, compassion, love and just a bit of playfulness; all the usual suspects, were proposed.

I then asked, "Given the nature of the group next week, how many of you will be attending?"

Eight hands went up. There were only two abstentions, one of the newcomers and Martha (phew).

I therefore established that next week's group was a "closed group" and that only today's eight volunteers could attend. Although it is delightful and optimum to have the same members of a group every week, the economics of running such groups works against this, as does the fluctuating pool of inpatients or day patients.

The following week as the group gathered there was a palpable sense of anticipation. There is an old maxim that the only difference between excitement and anxiety before any activity is the perception of whether you are going to cope or not. Excitement, I can cope! Fear, agh I'm not going to cope. Which is exactly the situation when my wife and I see a roller coaster: she gets very excited, I can't even look.

I was apprehensive as I sat down in group. How would this go? However, as always with a closed group, I had to trust the group. The group does the work. The group *holds* the group.

I ensured that the group were sat in a circle and that everyone could make direct eye contact with every other member.

I then started the group with a gentle check-in.

I asked the patient on my left to start the ball rolling by saying, "Given the agenda today, is shame how are you feeling?"

The consensus was that, yes, they were apprehensive but as one member said, "Oh shit, we just need to go where we don't want to go."

So, off we went.

I started by getting everyone to think about shame, their shame, what was it like?

The group quickly achieved consensus; shame was being defective, shame was about being dishonourable, shame was being bad.

Sam interrupted. "Shame is being disgusting."

The strength of her conviction stilled the group.

"Disgusting, because?"

"Because I am."

"Because?"

"Because I have done disgusting things."

"Because?"

"Because I needed heroin."

And then just when I was contemplating whether I could get away with a fourth "because," Jackie, the groups, most long serving member, said, "Last week you told us about how wonderful heroin was, but I was left wondering why you had such a powerful need for it?"

(Always let the group do the work).

Sam said, "Because when I was six I was sexually abused by a man across the road and when I told my mum she did not believe me. When I was thirteen, my dad, a long time alcoholic, died. My art teacher raped me and I went back and let him do it lots more until I got pregnant. My mother, a devout Catholic, threw me out of the house. So I stayed with an older male cousin, who in return for getting me an abortion, made me have sex with him. I was still at school and my cousin made me have sex with him every Friday night, in return for not charging me rent. By the time I was sixteen, I was charging his mates to have sex with me. That's why heroin was wonderful. All that shit went away."

Sam was staring ahead, her body rigid and defiant.

I said, "Sam watch this, feel this."

"Jackie," I said, "having heard what Sam has said, how do you feel about Sam?"

"I want to give her a hug."

In the group we have a strict guideline of no touching. You may aid a distressed member by passing the tissue box, but no physical contact. Mostly because it allows the toucher "off the hook" of their own ricocheted distress.

I invited each group member to likewise comment. All expressed similar sentiments of compassion, of acceptance, of empathy. One even said, "It's amazing you managed to ever give up heroin."

I noted to Sam, "Sam, you have just been bravely vulnerable. In doing so, what happened?"

Sam said with a sense of curiosity, "The group were not appalled, they seemed to understand."

I then asked each group member how Sam's story had impacted them. "Did they want to get closer to or further away from her?"

All said, "Closer."

"Yes," I said, "funnily enough, in being so vulnerable, so honest, you invited people in the group to come toward you. In trusting them with your vulnerability, they were able to get closer to you."

Sam sat quietly. I could see she was pondering.

WHAT HAPPENED?

There is a great question that I have unashamedly borrowed from Irvin Yalom. In one of his elegant clinical essays, he asked a client, "If you had been braver in session today, what would you have told me that you did not?"

It's one of those questions that you deploy at your own risk. The circumstances have to be right, the level of trust and safety for the person questioned has to high, the feeling tone of, in this case, the group has to be one of compassion, acceptance, curiosity and a bit of Anthony Storr's love. So I took a risk, asked the question, and the group, well, exploded.

"Sam, if you were really brave and took a chance, what might you now tell us that so far you have not?"

Sam looked at me, belligerently, defiantly. The group tensed. Had I pushed too far?

"Okay," she said, "you asked for it, you get it. When I was twenty-four I was very attractive."

Here she paused opened her handbag and passed around a photograph. She was right. The photograph was also a marker of the decaying physical impact of trauma.

"I was using lots of heroin and was working as a sex worker. I knew lots of the wrong people. I was made a proposition that if I took part in a series of porn movies I would be given free heroin."

"I did three movies; it was disgusting, it was degrading. Do you know that before you make a porn movie you have to put suppositories up your arse so that it's clean for them to use?"

The group is transfixed. Not a word is said.

"My porn movie name was Pixie. In one, I had sex with four men simultaneously. It was hideous. After I used up the heroin given to me, I never used again. Heroin wasn't worth doing that. I was better than that. But out there, somewhere, is my greatest shame, a porn movie titled, *Pixie Packs Them In*. It haunts me, I constantly look on the Internet to see if it's there, if everyone can see my shame."

Sam is sobbing, shaking, twitching and huddled over.

Jackie said, "I once had sex with three men at once, I just wanted to see if I could do it. I learned one thing from it, which is that you can't out fuck a woman. Sam, the heroes of porn are the women. They are the porn stars. The men are just animals. If we can cope with the sexual demands of various men, why we can cope with anything!"

Maisie, a Jewish South African woman of impeccable manners and posh domestic address went, "Ha, that's right. I've never told anyone but when I went back to university last year I met one of the security guards, and he's now my lover, and if I use speed I can have thirty or forty orgasms."

The room is alive; it's electric. Well, apart from the three men: me and the two male group members, we are quiet.

Then Aspeth, a former school principal, with a prodigious appetite for alcohol, gets in on the act. "Yes," she says, "it's a funny all the fuss made about sex. All those taboos about it. I once had sex, one at a time, in orderly sequence, with a whole football team."

Jackie jumped in, "What about the ones on the bench?"

"Oh yes," says Aspeth, with a grin, "I think I saved the worst to last."

There was laughter, energy, acceptance; a shared sense of "we will not be judged by our past sexual behaviour."

There was also a powerful sense of we are not our behaviour. An energetic discussion followed about not merging what we once did, with who we are.

Aspeth talked about her childhood in which she was constantly told she was a bad girl for behaving in certain ways. In the end she said she had internalised that she was bad. "That's why I drink," she said, "and they still tell me I'm bad."

Jackie then asked Sam, "If you heard the same story about being a sex worker and making porn movies from someone else here in the group, what would you say to them? What would you think of them?"

Sam answered, "I would tell them that I understand, that they were doing what they needed to do to survive. I would feel sorry for them and I would say, "Hey you are not what you do. There's not bad person in this room."

"Sam," I said, "but can you also let yourself off that hook of shame?"

She paused she said, "I don't know. I could forgive anyone else, but not me."

There's the trauma split.

Then to cap it all off, the female postgrad Clinical Psychology student sitting in on the group, said, "I've always wondered if I could be a porn star. I'm intrigued by how porn has changed the sexual landscape. I feel inadequate that my sex life is so ordinary. It's really, really boring."

"Sam, I know you were at your wit's end, but there's a bit of me that envies your experiences. At least you know about sex. I'm just so dull and uptight and being Pixie made you stop using heroin. If you hadn't been Pixie, you may be dead now."

Sam replied, "Yes, I sometimes allow myself a bit of breathing space and tell myself that Pixie saved me, but I usually jump on that quickly."

"Ah, you mustn't let yourself off that hook," I teased, "my goodness, whatever would happen if you did?"

Sam went quiet and queried, "I might just loathe myself less?"

"Absolutely."

Then out of nowhere the postgrad student said perceptively, "Sam, last week you said you were a wife, what happened?"

"Oh, I married Terry after I got clean. Funnily enough I met him in church. I used to go to church with mum, every now and then, to keep her company and sort of pretend I still believed. He was, like mum, a devout Catholic."

The Clinical Psych student asked, "Did you ever tell Terry about Pixie?"

"Good heavens, no." She said, "I told him I was a virgin. I made him wait for our wedding day."

The group roared with laughter.

Sam looked around at the laughing faces. When the noise subsided she simply said, "Thank you."

As she walked out of group that day she was taller.

The next week when group started, Sam said, "My agenda for today is to play a song I found that speaks for me, and maybe everyone in this room. I would like to have a bit of time to play my song."

The group needed no encouragement. Sam was "ordered" to immediately play her song. She got an Ipod and a speaker out of her bag and she handed out the lyrics to the Sia song "Alive."

The song is a telling, powerful, rebuttal of the shame of being abused.

The group spent the morning talking about Sam's song, Sia's song, about being survivors, and being alive, even if sometimes it meant "just breathing."

Augusten Burroughs is also a person to ask about shame. He wrote, "Shame is the *Doris* of emotions … Shame is a barnacle that you have to find, then scrape away. Shame is the reason why you feel less than, not enough, too much, or_____."

Chapter Twelve

You can't go past a vagina

Working with offenders has its own appeal and challenges. In my time, I have worked in three jails, two of them maximum security. Interestingly, as I started working in Glasgow, a paradigm for the management of very violent offenders was being established in the prison just down the road from our clinic. The idea was, you house the worst offenders together and let them (to a degree) look after themselves. The experiment that occurred in Barlinnie Prison has been copied worldwide.

I was thus intrigued some thirty years later, to be invited to consult in one such unit. As with the Barlinnie experiment, this was a unit within a maximum-security prison, having its own prison officers and its own way of being. The prisoners all classified as violent offenders also had their own "Violent Offenders Treatment Program."

My role was largely to work with a group of eight to ten offenders and explore with them the aetiology of drug use in their violent offending. The group was a psycho-educational one, so I had to lead the agenda; they filled in the content.

In working with this group, I quickly discovered that they utilised the concept that if they were drunk or intoxicated with methamphetamine or other stimulants, they couldn't help but be violent.

The drugs made them violent. I had a quick and ready response to this, which was, "Ah, so let me understand, when you're intoxicated you just can't help yourselves, you actually do things against your true natures?"

Usually the participants in this group leapt enthusiastically into the ambush I had set, "Too right doc, I just don't know what comes over me!" Or, "Doc, I'd never hurt a fly unless I was pissed." Or, "Too true doc, all of my violent offending has been meth-related."

Each group of offenders were largely in their mid-to-late forties and furiously, resolutely, heterosexual. "Ah," I'd say, "so sometimes when you get pissed or off your face on meth you might end up in bed with a man?"

Uproar would ensue. "Never doc!" "No way doc!" "That's disgusting!" "What's wrong with you doc? You queer?"

"Well," I'd go, "if alcohol or meth makes you go against your true natures, like being violent, why doesn't it make you queer? Clearly, as you have just stated, it is not in your natures to be violent or gay."

The universal answer was always, "But we're not like that!"

I'd agree. I'd say, "Yes, but you are violent. That *is* in your natures. So let's not make alcohol or meth the cause."

We'd then examine their violence and their childhoods.

When I did the PLACE exercise, the group would become silent and edgy. They all, always, scored below ten. They had all had childhood backgrounds of either being on the receiving end of violence, or from very early on, learnt that violence worked for them. Although for most of these offenders their violence was rage-based, for one or two, as with Mr. Smith, their violence was cool. They used violence as an instrument.

One such cool violent offender was Tony Merson. He was forty-seven, and physically very fit (aided and abetted by fourteen years of daily work-outs in the prison gym). He had a quiet authority and clearly, in a unit where power over the other was common currency, he was a top dog.

I always did an exercise in which I attempted to link what had happened to them in childhood with their current ways of being. I am of the opinion that it is important to understand why we are as we are. I would talk about personality and the impacts of growing up in a household where violence was a common occurrence.

As an interesting aside, at the time I was working in the prison, I was often invited by various organisations to run a workshop I had developed, called "Working with difficult and/or aggressive people."

I always started this workshop before it had actually started!

To explain: about five minutes before the workshop was scheduled to start, and as people were milling about chatting, finding a seat or being engrossed in their phones, I had an actor enter the workshop room. They would approach a pre-warned senior member of the group and literally start yelling abuse at the unfortunate manager. One actor got so into the role, and infuriated by the manager's efforts to appease her, she poured a jug of iced water over his head.

As soon as that happened I took charge of the group and shouted, "STOP."

The group literally froze. I then invited the group members to stay where they were and look around.

The impact of aggression has a hugely differential impact. As the group took stock of each other, they discovered some group members had disappeared under tables, some had run toward the doors, some had moved toward the altercation, and some were frozen to the spot. One or two were oblivious and still absorbed by their phones. Some were just gazing into space.

I would then get the participants into small groups to discuss why they had responded to the stooge incident in the way they did. Every time, it became quickly and readily apparent, that one's experience of aggression in childhood dictated how they responded.

On a personal note, on a recent trip to Jerusalem with my wife, there was a feeling of considerable tension following a series of stabbings. Armed military and police personnel were very evident.

As we walked around the Old Town, my wife was drawn to the bazaar and the myriad of shops. She was in her element. She was absorbed by the purchasing opportunities and especially taken by the place. After ten minutes or so of intense concentration, she turned to ask if I preferred tablecloth A or tablecloth B. I was fifty metres away with my back to a limestone cavern wall scrutinising every passer-by intently. I was on guard; she was blithely shopping.

We had very different childhoods, but funnily enough, both of us were enjoying ourselves.

When working with violent offenders it quickly becomes clear that most of them have a high level appreciation of the potential for violence. They seem to be able to sniff the air and detect it.

Early on in my career, I was at a research symposium where a psychology student, who doubled as a bar person at night, told how just before violence erupted in the pubs, there would be a pause, a lull, a chill. Glaswegians, she felt, were very good at sensing danger. At the time I wasn't persuaded. I am now.

With the violent offenders, I was keen to give them a sense of the possibility for change, but also some of the built in obstacles.

I knew that for many their very personalities were a problem.

Psychologists are a disagreeable lot. They bicker, argue and denounce each other, but when it comes to the nature of personality, they generally seem to agree.

One thing they agree on is that personality has five dimensions. A thing they are less certain about is the contribution of genetics to our personalities. However, I know precisely how much genetics affect our personality, because for about five years of my academic life, my office was right next to Professor David Hay who is a world authority on such matters. He said it was "thirty-five percent," so, thirty-five percent it is.

Below are the five components of personality that are thirty-five percent inherited.

WHAT HAPPENED?

When working with offenders I would stand before a white board and invite each of them to copy down what I wrote on the board.

(An important aside, if running a psychotherapeutic group, sit down. When running as in this case, a psycho-educational group, stand up).

I'd then draw a long line across the whiteboard. On the line I'd write "anxiety" and then at one end "LOW," the other "HIGH." I'd invite each of them to put a slash on their paper copy as to where they felt they landed on the high to low anxiety continuum. To demonstrate, I'd put a slash at about the seventy percent high mark as a measure of mine.

Then I'd draw another line. At one end I'd put "extrovert," the other "introvert." To assist, I'd add a few adjectives at each end like stimulus-hungry, easily bored, lots of friends, unreliable. At the other end retiring, a few close friends, reliable, likes to read.

Again I'd put a slash on the board for me, this time at about eighty percent extrovert.

The third line would be at one end, "open to new experiences, risk taker," the other end, "risk avoidant, closed to new experiences."

This time I'd slash at about the seventy percent risk accepting level.

Then a fourth line was "agreeable – disagreeable."

My slash would be somewhere left of the middle.

Finally, the fifth line would read "conscientious high – low."

My rating would be about ninety percent, to the high end.

I'd then get the participants to write their names on their self-rated personality scales and pass them around, so the group could see how they went in relation to others.

What always surprised them was that they were so much alike.

- High on extraversion
- Low on anxiety
- High on open to new experiences
- Low on agreeableness … and
- Low on conscientiousness.

Unfortunately, a mix of personality dimensions that invited trouble.

Their personalities predisposed them to being fearless, stimulus-hungry, unreliable risk takers who were low on agreeableness and conscientiousness. All the backdrop characteristics of so-called "anti-social personality disorder."

I'd then take the discussion a bit further and tell them, from the discussions we had about their childhoods in which I considered there was "too much of the wrong stuff and not enough of the right stuff," their childhood would probably have had some impact on their current functioning.

Most of them told of how they had to fend for themselves, of how using power over others was preferable to being vulnerable. One day on a bit of a whim, I asked each member of the group to define "masculinity." After much intense debate, Tony Merson jumped up took the white board marker from my hand, and led the group to consensus. He wrote on the board:

"Masculinity is about being SELF RELIANT, being in CONTROL, maintaining your POWER over others and, if you have to, use VIOLENCE."

The group sat back satisfied. The sense was, "Yes, that's it, that's a real man."

Until Tony said, with a shake of his head, "But, that's the fucking reason why we're all in here."

So they turned to me and said, "So what is masculinity, Bill?"

"Ah well," I go, "that depends who you ask."

I told them that, in preparation for the group, I had asked a male friend, a female patient and my wife.

I ran the definitions past them, starting with that of my friend.

"Masculinity is having a hairy chest, and wearing shorts and a tee shirt all year round."

A big hirsute biker said, "That's me, I qualify." The group laughed.

Next, the female patient's definition:

"Masculinity is about being a provider, a protector and also being able to hold the baby."

The group went quiet.

"So, how's about your missus?" Questioned one group member.

"Masculinity is about being able to see when I hurt, to stop and listen to me."

Complete silence, until one offender broke the uncomfortableness with:

"So, doc, it's official then, you are queer."

Raucous laughter to cover their disquiet.

The saddest thing about working with violent offenders is that inside they know they don't really measure up. They know they've had compassion beaten out of them.

This became very evident whenever I'd draw a big triangle on the whiteboard. At the top of the triangle I'd write "TRUST," bottom left "EMOTIONAL VULNERABILITY," and bottom right "INTIMACY."

The group would always look questioningly at me. "What's that about, doc?"

"Well," I'd say, "most of us want connection to others. Intimacy, boys, is not sex, it is connection. It's about having a relationship with someone who has your back. It's about having someone in your life with who you can share your darkest fears and deepest worries, where you can just be your undefended self."

"But," I continued, "if you want intimacy, you have to be prepared to show your emotional vulnerability. You need to test out the other person by telling them a bit about your vulnerability and seeing whether they can be trusted with your secret concerns."

As I was speaking I'd draw a series of arrows starting from Emotional Vulnerability and moving toward Trust. "If you offer a bit of your vulnerable self to another and they are compassionate and listen (and don't laugh or run off and tell others what you said), then you can learn to trust someone emotionally. And the more you emotionally trust them, the closer you become, the more intimacy you have, and then you can be more emotionally vulnerable."

In the group I would always see complete and utter disbelief.

For them the triangle was an alien world. In the childhoods of the violent offender cohort, the lesson, of course, was don't be vulnerable, don't trust, remain detached, be self-reliant; always use whatever you have to remain in control, use power over, and violence if you need to, but never, ever, be emotionally vulnerable. If you are, then you will be exploited.

Beneath the machismo, the aggressive posturing, away from the "leave me alone" warnings of the beards, big muscles and tattoos, deep inside and shuttered off in childhood, violent offenders yearn for what they never got. They yearn for connection; so they belong to bikie clubs, or right wing supremacist groups, crime gangs or drug cartels.

As a therapist with such damaged individuals, your capacity to connect and get alongside them as vulnerable individuals is the only corrective curative hope they have.

I have always liked what is known as "deterrence theory." Basically, in deterrence theory, it is posited that what makes people conform, is not their inherent goodness, but their perception of whether they will get caught.

Thus, it's not the *actual* risk of being caught, but the *perception* of the likelihood of being caught. Interestingly, work on deterrence theory shows that having the death penalty for drug smuggling is not a deterrent. Severity of punishment doesn't matter because people inclined to drug deal/smuggle have the actual experience of getting away with it; often on a daily basis. They know that the odds of getting caught are very, very low.

Unfortunately it's often the naive and anxious drug mules who get caught and executed.

So I'd say to the group, "Imagine this. Your daughter babysits for the family up the road. One night, while poking about in the house, she discovers a big box in a back bedroom filled with bank notes of various denominations. She excitedly reports there must be at least a quarter of a million in there!"

I continue. "She also tells you that the family are going away for four days next week and she has been invited to go with them to act as a live-in baby sitter. Can she go?"

"Of course, she can!"

"Now then boys, that's two hundred and fifty thousand just sitting there waiting; in all probability, in untraceable banknotes."

I then would say, "Now, if your chance of getting caught nicking the dosh is one in ten thousand, would you do it? If yes, put your hands up."

Inevitably, never mind the size of the group, all hands would excitedly go up.

I dropped the odds of capture.

"One in five thousand."

All the hands are still up.

As the odds of getting caught dropped, so would a few hands. Usually, by the time it got to one in one hundred, half the group would have opted out. Deterrence theory works.

"One in fifty?" Another hand may decline the adventure.

By "one in ten" there were always just two or three left.

"One in five?" Two left

"One in two." One left

"One in one." One left.

I'd always say, "One in one means you are going to get caught!"

And the one left would say something like, "You can't let that money just sit there!"

I never really understood that. Maybe deterrence theory isn't quite right.

Tony Merson was one of the ones who left his hand up.

After I'd run my six or so sessions, Tony approached me in a break and asked if it would be possible for me to see him individually?

I explained that I was only contracted to run groups. However, Tony said he would arrange for me to be paid as a private psychologist. With permission from the prison authorities, once a month after my group session I saw Tony individually.

I explored with him his childhood. A drunken, violent father and a drug-dependent mother. The middle of three boys, Tony told me that from the off, he always got into trouble. Even in primary school, he constantly absented himself and went off on his own exploring. He shoplifted, he graffiti-ed, he fare-dodged on trains and buses, he did a few breaking and entering's. He said by the time he was in high school he was unable to tolerate the frustrations of not knowing what was really happening in class. Barely able to read or write and hopeless with maths, he quickly became a drug dealer. He made links with some serious criminals. He started to prosper.

He told me with no remorse that his dad had come home drunk and belligerent one day, and had then proceeded to beat him for not going to school. Tony said he waited until his father was asleep and then set fire to the house. It literally burnt to the ground.

WHAT HAPPENED?

There is an old adage about arson, which is "burnt children burn." And they usually burn down the house, school or orphanage where they were abused.

One patient told me as a ten year old, she witnessed her father murder her mother, for which he was subsequently imprisoned. She was taken into care in a local Roman Catholic orphanage. Here she was repeatedly sexually abused by the priests and physically abused by the nuns. She said, in a flat, eyeless, calm voice, "When I was fourteen I burnt the orphanage down."

I said, without pause, "Well done."

Tony said by the time he was nineteen he had a black V8 ute, money and two guns. He augmented his drug dealing income by contracting his muscle out as an enforcer. Inflicting pain did not worry him: "Weak pricks should pay their bills."

At age twenty-one he was involved in armed robbery in which a security guard was run over and killed. Although not the driver, Tony was deemed to be an accessory and was sentenced to nine years imprisonment.

On his release he quickly re-established himself as drug dealer and enforcer. He and a mate decided that a local bank was an ideal venue for a hold up. Unfortunately, as Tony laughingly said, he was so hyped up on a mixture of adrenalin and speed that on entering the bank, he completely forgot to lower the visor of his motorcycle helmet. Two days later, his grinning, wide-eyed face was on the front page of the local newspaper. He was arrested, literally fleeing to the border.

It was this offence for which he was currently imprisoned. He was due for parole and I suspected (rightly), that part of his wish to see me privately was to make a good impression. However, he was, underneath the bravado of his offending, concerned that unless he managed things differently, he would inevitably end up inside again.

So we put in place a deal, if he got parole I would see him regularly on the outside and we would focus on his impulsivity and acceptance of risk. I reminded him he was the only person in a group of violent offenders who had said he'd "do it anyway" even if it was certain he would get caught. He smiled and acknowledged he had things to learn.

Some six months later he came to see me. For the next four months he was a regular, twice-a-month attender.

I enjoyed seeing him. He was an articulate storyteller and quietly charming and charismatic. He appeared to be giving the straight world a go. He had a job as a concreter and although he said the pay was "shit," it left him too tired at night to get into too much mischief. Usefully, several of his former criminal contacts were incarcerated.

I reminded him of his predilection to do wrong things even though he was bound to get caught. I asked him to explain what that was about. I told him that I didn't understand it.

Then he told me this.

"Ha, Bill it's like this. Last week I was out with my girlfriend. We'd hired a limo so we could have a drink on the way into town. We'd booked dinner at Maestros and then went to a club. I'd taken some speed so I was drinking a bit and having fun. At about 2am my girlfriend said she wanted to go home, so I called the limo guy and arranged for him to pick us up. But, you know Bill, I wasn't quite done. I wanted more. I had this energy."

"As we were being driven home it was pouring down. I spotted this girl walking home. She was drenched. So I asked the driver to pull over and see if she was heading our way."

He continued, "As she climbed into the car I saw she was very fit. I asked her where she was heading, but it was not on our route home, in fact it was miles away. So I said to her that if she had sex with me, I'd get her dropped to her door."

"And, Bill, she agreed. It was great fun."

He paused. "My girlfriend's left me though."

I said, "So why do it?"

"Because," he said with a gleam in his eye, "Bill, in this life you must never go past a vagina."

I graphically understood him. The hallmark feature of impulsivity coupled with a total lack of concern about consequences was explained. For him, and for some other offenders, missing an opportunity is far worse than getting caught.

If as a child you got nothing, anything, *whatever the consequences,* is better than nothing.

There is now evidence from brain scans that some people when offered a reward have much higher activity in the dopamine reward centre than others. The more "psychopathic" you are, the more likely you are to have a brain that acts this way. This has prompted a "dysfunction in the dopamine brain reward circuitry" hypothesis for people like Tony.

However, just because two things go together, it does not mean that one causes the other. Take the interesting issue of storks and babies. In Sweden, the number of stork nests in urban areas is, on most counts, about four times higher than in rural areas. Impressively, the number of live human births in urban Sweden is about four times higher than in rural areas. Voila, storks deliver babies.

It is equally possible that the noted brain differences between more psychopathic and less psychopathic individuals are a consequence of trauma in childhood. If you have a childhood in which you constantly miss out on getting any of the right stuff, and too much of the wrong stuff, then access to anything that looks like "the right stuff" would be very appealing and far more irresistible than to those that have the early childhood experience of having lots of the right stuff.

Some three months later Tony stopped coming to see me. He had been arrested driving a Ferrari with five kilos of methamphetamine in the boot. The car wasn't his, and of course, he didn't know about the drugs in the boot. He was just helping a mate out delivering a car to Adelaide. He was sentenced to nine years. It must have been simply irresistible.

I hate to admit it, but I think some people are so damaged in their childhoods that even psychotherapy may not be enough to rectify the wounds of the past.

Chapter Thirteen
Addiction doesn't exist

One of the most gratifying aspects of being a psychotherapist is to work with someone at the brink and travel with them to stability.

As British psychologist Dorothy Rowe has so elegantly articulated: "A good therapist is one who knows that the task of the therapist is to accompany the client on a journey without maps to an unknown destination where, on reaching it, the client will know it for the first time."

My first meeting with Sarah was not encouraging, not encouraging at all.

A day earlier I had had an email from a psychiatric colleague:

"Bill, can you see Sarah Taylor. I admitted her yesterday. She's probably the world's oldest methamphetamine user. She's sixty, very paranoid, hostile and crazy. Good luck. Dr. P."

Forewarned is forearmed, so the next day during a break in running an in-patient group, I went to the ward, checked her room number, and asked the nursing staff, "How's Mrs. Taylor?"

I was told she hadn't come out of her room since her admission.

So I duly went and knocked on her door. A growl invited me in. The room was almost pitch black and the smell was hot and fetid.

I never got to introduce myself. "Who the fuck are you?"

"I'm Bill Saunders. Dr. P has asked me to see you."

"I don't want to see anyone. I don't want to be here. I want to go home."

I am a great believer in matching my language to that of the patient. Having trained in Glasgow, where fuck is a noun, a verb, a gerundive, an adverb, an adjective and an all-round most useful word, swearing doesn't bother me at all.

Once when working in England I had a laptop that imploded. I took it urgently to the computer shop on the corner. The technician just happened to be a Glaswegian. He told me to come back in an hour; he'd have a diagnosis by then. On my anxious return his diagnosis didn't please me, but his choice of words did. "The fucking fucker's, fucking, fucked." Brilliant.

However, some practitioners working in mental health are offended by "bad" language. For example, once after giving a university sponsored public lecture I was upbraided by a fellow academic who chastisingly said, "Bill, do you think your language was appropriate, there was a nun in the room?"

I'd actually used the word "fuck" in a quote from a patient who said delightfully about his relapse: "Bill, I knew what was going to happen when I bought the bottle of vodka. I knew I would drink the whole bottle and then go on a bender, but just for once I was hoping that this time it would turn out fucking different."

A clever comment, a reflective comment and one definitely worthy of a "fuck" in it. Ever since, I have repeated that quote in numerous groups where alcohol and drug dependent clients have nodded sagely. One even perspicaciously said, "Yes, it's the hope that kills you."

So, my view about bad language is that if you, as a nurse, psychologist, doctor, group worker, counsellor or nun, get offended by bad language, then you are in the wrong fucking job.

But, back to Sarah Taylor.

"Yes," I said, "it really fucks to be in a place like this, doesn't it?"

"Yes, it fucking does," she said. "It's shit. Now who are you?"

"I'm Bill Saunders, I'm a Clinical Psychologist." I got no further.

"What the fuck's that?"

"Ha," I said smiling, "good question. I'm someone your psychiatrist thinks it might be useful for you to talk to. Dr. P will manage your medication and your stay here and I'm available, if you wish, to be your therapist."

She thought for the moment.

Then said, "So what the fuck are your credentials for being my therapist?"

Ah, another great question and a telling question. I avoided the trap of saying "Well, I've got a Masters and a PhD," and instead said:

"What do you want to know about me, so that you can trust me?"

For the next fifteen minutes, in that gloomy, hot, fetid room we started that essential process of psychotherapy; developing trust.

By the end I managed to coax her into allowing me to open the blinds, turn on the air conditioning and then bring her a cup of tea and a cake from the kitchen. We agreed we could try some talking therapy. From humble beginnings great things can be achieved.

Much fuss is made about addiction; drug addiction, shopping addiction, sexual addiction, cocaine addition, Facebook addiction, methamphetamine addiction, Internet addiction, *Game of Thrones* addiction, the most addictive drug in the world addiction, and so on. It's all nonsense: nonsense, because addiction does not exist.

If you are not persuaded by that assertion consider the following precis of a story by Stephen King entitled *Quitters Inc.*

In this short story, a man visits a smoking cessation clinic. He hands over $2000 and is told that in a year he will be abstinent.

He laughs, leaves the clinic and has a cigarette. Twenty minutes later his phone rings. His wife is screaming in agony. She says that two guys entered the house and without saying a word, cut off, with a bolt cutter, the little finger of her left hand.

He's rushing home when his phone rings again. It's the clinic. He's told, "You have a choice, you can continue to smoke, but every time you do your wife will lose another finger, or you can stop smoking and your wife will keep her remaining fingers."

In Stephen King's story, the central character stops smoking. A year later he attends a clinic arranged, "one-year-straight" celebration. His wife is also invited. When he shakes the hands of the spouses of the other successful quitters, they all have fingers missing, some several.

I have over the years used the message of Stephen King's story in a variety of ways. One I remember was both satisfying and effective. I was running a group when one member, a recently admitted, loud, aggressive and dominating methamphetamine user, when asked to introduce himself, said, "My name's Steve and I'm addicted to meth."

I just couldn't help myself. "Steve, how do you know you're addicted?"

"I can't stop, doc!"

"You can't stop, because?"

"Because, I'm addicted, Doc."

"How do you know you're addicted, Steve?"

"Because I can't stop," said Steve tetchily.

"We're going round in circles, Steve," I said, "just like your drug use."

Then I deployed Stephen King's wisdom.

"Steve, who do you love even more than yourself?"

(As an aside, from a psychological perspective the right answer is "no one," but I've only ever heard that once).

Steve thinks and says, "My mum."

"Ok Steve," I said, "now here's a deal. You pay me $2000 and I guarantee you, you will get straight."

Steve goes, "Yeah right," in disbelief. I pretend to take the fee off him.

"Okay Steve, now it gets real simple. Because of my job I know some bikies. They occasionally do errands for me, especially when I pay them a thousand dollars. If you ever use speed again (and as of now you will be urine tested randomly and repeatedly) I will get those bikies to visit your mum. They will rape her, they will sodomise her and then they will cut off a finger and bring it back as a souvenir for you!" I always felt Stephen King's intervention needed a bit more bite, after all we are talking about drug "addiction."

Steve looks around the room aghast. Defiant, he says, "What you can't do that!"

"Actually I can," I say, "but the question is Steve, what are you going to do?"

"Fuck," he said, "of course, if I knew that was really going to happen I'd stop."

"So what does that say about your relationship with meth, Steve?"

It slowly dawned on Steve that he'd been ambushed.

"Fuck," he says, "it says that if things got really bad like that then I would stop."

Caitlin Thomas, the wife of the writer Dylan Thomas wrote in her autobiography, *Double Drink Story*, that at one stage in his life, Dylan Thomas was confronted with a choice about alcohol.

She wrote, "He could drink and die, or get sober and live. He chose to drink and he died."

She continued, "Some years later I was confronted with the exact same choice. I could drink or live. I chose to live."

Then she added, "I keep wondering if I made the right choice."

Ah, well you get that, post-decisional regret it's called, or buyer's remorse.

The word addiction is like a number of other words (lazy or "not motivated" are other good examples) that are literally intervening variables of no explanatory value. The statement "I'm addicted" is determined by not being able to stop that in turn defines addiction. A tautology that excuses and permits the behaviour.

The word addiction comes from the Latin verb *addicere,* to enslave. In Roman times if you owed Caesar money you were "enslaved" to him. You literally had to be his slave until you paid off your debt and then, and only then, would he let you free. Your freedom was his choice not yours. You had no choice, well, other than death. But drug dependence is totally different because you can always choose to stop.

People play the addiction card because as Prof. John Booth Davies wrote in his seminal book, *The Myth of Addiction,* it makes everyone, doctors, addicts, friends and lovers, and others, "happy." It's much better to believe your partner is trying their best, but their addiction got them, rather than they relapsed because they wanted to.

My experience is that dependent drug users, alcohol users, or gamblers, love to make things complicated. The more complicated things are the more reasons they have to continue. My response is clear.

I say, "Guys, this is not rocket science. This "addictions" thing is very simple. You either," (and I stretch out one arm to the side) "decide to stop, or," (and I stretch out my other hand to the other side) "or you decide to continue. Both are choices. Both are tough choices. Choosing to stop is tough and choosing to continue will be tough. So make your choice and stick with it."

You can't choose whether to have cancer or not. However much you may dislike it, hate it, want it gone, you can't will it away. However, if you are dependent on any drug or behaviour such as gambling, you can always wake up one day and say, "I'm not doing this anymore." To reiterate: being dependent on drug use is not a disease, or an addiction, it is a choice.

Many years ago, I was undertaking some research into the drinking habits of people living in the west of Scotland. A coincidental finding was that a cohort of respondents acknowledged that, yes they used to drink too much in the past, but no longer did so. So we went back and re-interviewed this sub-sample of some 190 individuals. What we discovered surprised me.

The first surprise was that the overwhelming majority had changed their drinking behaviour without any professional help. The second was that even very entrenched drinkers gave almost "trivial" reasons for so doing.

One respondent, a bottle-of-scotch-a-day man, reported that he had gone to his favourite pub for a drink when the barman started talking about the new car he had just bought. The respondent said, "I thought he's buying that car with my money. What have I got?" He finished his drink, walked out of the pub and never drank again.

Interestingly, the literature is now replete with such examples across all types of drug use. Giving up your drug use is a choice.

Thus, therapy for people with so-called addiction problems is really straightforward. You have to organise it so they say to themselves, "I don't want to do this anymore."

This, of course, involves motivation of the "shall I or shan't I?" type.

For anyone who has an entrenched dependence of any substance or behaviour, it is always necessary to "clear the decks for action." That is, the drug dependence has to be addressed before the underlying reasons for using so excessively are addressed. I was from the outset suspicious of Sarah's childhood, but first things first, could I invoke Sarah to persuade herself (probably against her will) to choose to become abstinent?

Although the following is a fictional account of my motivational intervention with Sarah, I know it is a fictional version that is based on fact. Also in our later work, Sarah often reiterated the facts relating to her stopping and how one session of psychotherapy was, in her words, "life-saving."

As an aside, some months later when teaching GPs about motivation, I used

WHAT HAPPENED?

Sarah as a live client in a clinical demonstration where she literally pretended to be a recently admitted patient with an active methamphetamine problem. In effect I got to do the interview with Sarah twice.

It is important to note, I only deploy my motivational intervention when I have established a good therapeutic alliance with a client.

"Sarah," I said, "may I focus for a bit on your methamphetamine use?"

"Yes."

"Thanks. Okay now, what for you are the best, good things about meth?"

Sarah's response was very quick.

"I love the hit, the feel of the needle, the rush, the bliss."

"Other good things?"

"Yes," more thoughtfully, "I love the sense of relief, the tension goes, I feel better."

I prompted, "Better?"

"Yes better, much better, the self-loathing, the hatred goes. I feel better about me, better about the world. It's just so much fucking better."

"Any other good things about meth?"

"No, that's about it, coming off is total shit though."

"Yes, I'm sure, but let me recap the good things."

I had furiously scribbled down everything she said. Although I don't normally take notes in therapy, when doing a motivational interview I always take comprehensive notes. It is very important that the client hears back *exactly* what they have said, *in their own words.*

This is because there is a psychological law that pertains directly to motivation It is, "I learn what I believe as I hear myself speak."

Okay, if you are feeling a little let down by this psychological law, email Prof. Bill Miller at the University of Albuquerque in New Mexico, because it's his law. However, just think about it a bit. How good is this law really? What does it tell us?

Well, first it tells us never to argue with anyone, because "they learn what they believe as they hear themselves speak." I have to say I have never seen anyone (myself included) say, after arguing with someone for while, "Well, bugger me, you are totally right, I've been talking nonsense."

It just doesn't happen, does it? Why not? Because of the psychological law "I learn what I believe a I hear myself speak."

Importantly, so do clients. The way to get patients to motivate themselves is to let them hear themselves. Let them hear what they really think about themselves and, as in this case, their drug use.

So I repeated back to Sarah what she had told me.

"For you the good things about meth are that you love the hit, the feel of the needle, the rush, the bliss, and that you love that sense of relief when the tension goes and you feel better, because your self-loathing and hatred goes. Also the world as a whole becomes a much fucking better place."

She nodded and said, "That's it, that's why I love the stuff!"

I said, "Yes, I can see that it has a very powerful attraction for you. However, if we may, can we flip the coin over and can you tell me what *for you* are the less good things about your meth use?"

(Always *less good* never bad - less good reels them in). Having asked the good question first, I've already lured them into a debate that at the front end looks even handed (good v less good), but the whole process is actually a psychological ambush.

Sarah mulled over the question; she took her time, but once she started a torrent of nasties poured out.

"Well, to start there is the cost, then there is the paranoia, sometimes I don't even know I'm paranoid. Do you know I thought the police were after me, when I drove up to the hospital. I counted forty-three police cars, strangely, some of them were orange, do they have orange cars?"

She continued, "Then there's the fact that I don't sleep and that makes me more crazy and I do things that I wouldn't normally do. Last week I fucked an electrician who came to the house to fix the air con. I offered him me rather than cash. I needed the cash to score. But, I also go on shoplifting binges to pay for it. I do all sorts of things to pay for it. Then you have to score and that can take ages. Then it's fucking groundhog day, steal, score, use, steal, score, use, steal, score, use." She paused, I waited.

"I've let my children down. They won't let me babysit anymore because I'm too angry, too unreliable. I fall asleep when I should be minding their kids. I'm wasting my fucking life. I'm trapped. I can't stop. I need to stop. I must stop. I can't stop. It's a nightmare. I hate meth." She started crying.

Now this is when a novice motivational interviewer may buckle. They may hand over a tissue, offer an empathic conjecture, seek to soothe.

Don't. Keep the pressure building, so here is some psychological pus, ramp it up. Remain detached, unperturbed; this is the first part of the kill.

"So, Sarah," I say, and read back her words to her. "The less good things about meth for you are:
the cost
the paranoia
the not knowing whether you're paranoid
orange police cars
lack of sleep
becoming more crazy

fucking electricians to save some cash to score with
shoplifting
the scoring
the repetition
every day is ground hog day
letting down your kids
not being allowed to be grandma
the wanting to stop
not being able to stop
the need to stop
knowing you must stop
but you don't."
She nodded resignedly.
"Other less good things?" I prompt (people never tell you the worst bits first time).
"Isn't that fucking enough?" Sarah asked. I sensed her reluctance to go further.
So a nudge, "What are the other less good things?"
She literally whimpered, "I get very frightened, I think there are people in my house, I think I'm going to get raped again, I have to bolt myself in the house and when I go out I have three padlocks to stop people getting in while I'm out. I hear things, I have a voice telling me I'm crap, I have voice telling me to watch out, that people are out to get me. Last month the voice told me my daughter was going to dob me in about shoplifting." She paused. "I got so mad, scared crazy mad, that I stabbed her."
She sat and wailed.
I didn't let up; this agony, this emotional ocean of pus, is the heart of change.
"Now Sarah, so you have voices in your head, you become very frightened, you think you're going to be raped again and last month you became so crazy mad that you stabbed your daughter?"
She nodded dejectedly.
I show her the long list of "less good" things.
"Which one of these less good things concerns you most?"
Through her tears she looked at the list.
"Fucking obvious isn't it, I'm a mad, old, dangerous cunt."
I nodded in agreement.
I appeared to change tact, but I'm just maneuvering to turn the screw a little tighter.
"Sarah, part of you is a mad old cunt, but tell me tell me about that other Sarah, your best-self Sarah? What might a good friend, or your daughters say were your best qualities?"

(My experience is that if you ask directly, first person, "what are your good qualities?" then most dependent drug users will tell you they don't have any, but in third person mode they can struggle up a response).

Sarah thought. She replied haltingly.

"Well, my daughter used to tell me I was a great mum." She stalled.

"Great, because?"

Sarah thought, shook her head, "Because in the past, she could rely on me."

She stopped and then more forcefully got in touch with her past self.

"I was compassionate, I was thoughtful, I can be funny, I was good at getting out of scrapes, I was patient, I was kind, I was okay, … but, not anymore."

I then invited her to see her as the drug dependent person, but used her language. "Okay, then, let's hear about that other you? Let's hear about the drug dependent crazy old cunt, what words would you use about her?"

This is much easier. It poured out.

"She's despicable, a lying shite, she's dishonest, crazy, mean, angry, vicious violent, horrible, selfish, jealous, crazy with voices in her head. She's a bad mad cunt."

She stopped. She was sobbing

I held out my left hand. "Sarah, look at me, this hand is good you."

I repeat her words, "This you is a great mum, reliable, compassionate, funny, thoughtful, good at getting out of scrapes, kind, patient."

I held out my right hand, "This is dependent you, the crazy, mad cunt you, that is despicable, a lying dishonest shite, who's crazy, mean, angry, vicious, violent, horrible, selfish, jealous, crazy with voices in her head, a mad cunt."

Sarah stared at my hands. "How do these two 'yous' go together?"

She whispered through her pain, "They don't, they don't go together at all."

"How does that feel?"

"It feels terrible."

"Because?"

"Because, fuck, because I've lost me, I'm fucking lost."

"Because?"

"Because I'm not being me." (Gotcha).

"Because?" (That's the three).

"Because of fucking meth." She is wracked by sobs.

I pounce.

"Do you think you will be using meth in five years' time?"

"No."

"Four years' time?"

"No."

"Three years?"

WHAT HAPPENED?

"No!"
"Two years' time?"
"No! No!"
"One years' time?"
"For fuck's sake, no! No! No! No!"
"Next week?"
She stopped and looked up, "You bastard," she said.
I smiled.
"Okay, okay, no. Not next week, not ever."
I then turned the screw.
"So *what* are you going to do about your meth use?"
Quietly, "I'm going to stop."
I just can't help it, "because?"
"Because I'm lost, because I can't win, because I want to be me."
"So what *are* you going to do about your meth use?"
"I'm going to do whatever you say is a good thing to do. I will listen, I will surrender, I will stop."
I said gently, "So Sarah let me hear what are *you* going to do about your meth use?"
"I'm going to put it behind me, I'm going to crawl my way back, I'm going to make amends, I'm going to find the real me."
I stopped the interview.

Today Sarah is ten years straight. That day was the beginning of a long journey. You always have to see beyond the substance, but you cannot do that if you are drowning in it.

So Sarah got herself off meth. For the next two years we explored what had happened to her to make her be like this. It was a long painful and horrible story. It was a story of childhood neglect and shocking physical and sexual abuse. Over time she also gave up alcohol, cannabis, cigarettes, pain pills, shoplifting, random electricians and hearing voices.

Every Christmas I get a card and an update. The last one just said:

"I'm alive and well and being a beautiful grandma. Keep on being a cunt to us junkies."

To cite the late, very brilliant and much missed, Prof. John Booth Davies: "Motivation is not stuff you can put into people. They have to find it for themselves."

Chapter Fourteen
Must get it right

Traumatic abusive childhoods can be double-edged swords. They clearly instil emotional dysregulation and other personal demons, but may also bestow some virtues. Dr. Mae Liu was a case in point.

She made the referral herself, she phoned and insisted that "no one must know." She even stipulated that she had to attend under an assumed name. So she became Dr. Mae Liu and even my case notes were in that alias. Mental health disorders are stigmatising and ironically no where more so than in medicine. She said she had diagnosed herself as having an "anxiety disorder."

On presentation Dr. Liu was petite, elfin, immaculate, *and* very distressed. She looked younger than her thirty-two years and as she sat neatly on the sofa in my office, it was difficult to see her as anything but a young woman who was out of her depth, drowning.

She answered my "what brings you to see a psychologist" question by stating, "I'm a paediatric registrar at the children's hospital. In two months I am going to sit my college membership entrance examination and I'm terrified I'm going to fail."

"Because?"

"Because it's a hard exam with a seventy percent failure rate. And I just cannot fail. I have to pass, but I'm so anxious about failing that I can't concentrate on studying. All I can think about is that F."

"Mae," I said, "I'm very curious, help me understand something. You are a doctor, you have sat and obviously passed many exams, so why is this exam so terrifying for you?"

Mae paused and said, "I've always been anxious about examinations, but this one is really big. This one determines whether I make it or don't make it."

"Make it?"

"Yes, make it. Listen, my father is a consultant surgeon, my mother is a professor of English, my older brother is a consultant cardiologist, and my little sister has a PhD from Harvard and is an assistant professor in Singapore. You see I cannot fail. But I know I'm going to. My family will be shamed. We do not fail."

I felt overwhelmed by the intensity of all of this achievement.

"Your family feels overwhelming."

Mae reprimanded me and said what was perspicaciously true, "I've lived with them all my life, well, until I recently got married and even then we lived with them for a while, so I don't know any different. I'm used to them."

"Yes, of course, sorry, tell me about growing up in this family of yours, what was it like?"

I had an image of a red hot, intense crucible in my head, but Mae's reflections were different. Her delivery was interestingly staccato, devoid of warmth. I wondered whether she was repeating learned lines.

"It was good. It was very ordered. I liked that. Because dad worked long hours we didn't see too much of him, but mum, even though she was studying for her PhD, she was always there when we came in from school. She would make us afternoon tea then my siblings and I would go to our study room and do our homework together. We had to study for two hours each night. It was hard, boring, but was very good training for medical school. After supper my siblings and I played the musical instruments we were learning. My brother played the guitar, I played the piano and my sister played the violin. Sometimes dad would listen to us play. Mum was our music teacher; she was very strict, we had to practice every day, but it worked. I now love playing the piano, it's a favourite pastime."

"And, at the weekends?" I prompted.

"It was the same," said Mae. "In the mornings mum would set us homework and then in the afternoons we would practice our music. On Saturday nights we would visit mum's family for dinner and on Sunday, dad's. We had to, what is that English expression?" she said. I looked at her quizzically. "Ah yes," she said almost proudly, "we had to be seen, but not heard."

"How about friends?"

"We were allowed friends at school, but they were never invited to the house. Mum said friends can get in the way of learning. I had one friend all the way through school, but I lost touch with her when I came here to study medicine."

I was curious given the imposed external structure of her childhood how Mae had coped with being "a free spirit" student at an Australian medical school.

"So how was the transition from home to university for you?"

"It was good," said Mae, "my brother came to university here first, and mum got her aunt to come over and he lived with her and she looked after him. Then when I also got a scholarship here, mum took a sabbatical for a year, and we all lived together. It worked well, mum put in place exactly the same structure as at home."

Mae paused, "You know," she said, "it always amazed me that the local medical students passed their exams, they all seemed to be going to parties, getting drunk and never studying. I supposed they must have done though."

"Mae, where is mum now?"

"She's back in Singapore, has been for the last three years."

I expressed surprise, "Oh, I thought she had only stayed for your first year at university?"

Mae apologised, "Sorry, I didn't tell you my mother got a job teaching at the same university that my brother and I were studying at and then my little sister studied here before going to the States to do her PhD in physics. Mum used to make a joke that she should have got a degree in medicine and in physics because she coached us all, all the way through uni."

"How does it feel, Mae, not to have your mum here to help you with this exam?"

Mae looked at her feet. "Terrifying, I've never passed an exam without mum's help, I owe her everything, I'm not sure I can do it without her."

Herein was the crux. Parents who exert external control over their children deny them self-control. You can't learn self-control other than by being given the opportunity to get out of control. And there was another matter.

"Mae, tell me about failing this exam? What would it mean?"

"It would mean I'm not good enough, that I'm a failure, that I'm not enough. I can't fail this exam."

She started to cry, she wailed. "I'm not studying enough to pass."

Her distress was palpable. It was extreme, it was too much, too disorganised, and therein was the answer.

I let her settle.

"Tell me, Mae, if you fail this exam, can you take it again?"

"Oh, yes I think you can have three or four attempts. My brother failed his Royal College of Surgeons' exam twice before he got through."

"Ah, so you could fail it and then do it again."

She reacted with a rebuke. "I cannot fail this exam. You do not understand." She sat and cried.

But I thought I did, when people over-react, when an event assumes disproportionate meaning, when someone's distress at a possible outcome is so palpable that it feels overwhelming then it is an echo, an echo of past trauma; a marker of something very bad happening way back when.

I said, "Mae, tell me about failing exams in the past, what happened?"

WHAT HAPPENED?

She sat mute. She shuddered. She said, in a low, small voice, "I would be beaten. My mother bought canes in the market to beat me. I had to get seventy percent or better on all my tests. She had the school send all my results to her, even for inconsequential classroom tests. For every percentage point under seventy percent I would get one hit with the cane. One day I got to school and I thought that I had a physics test coming up, but I got it wrong. The test was chemistry. I got forty-five percent.

"When my mother got the result she made me undress and stand in front of her. I was thirteen. She took six new canes out of a pack and thrashed me. She whipped me twenty five times. She counted them out. She told me I wasn't as clever as my brother or my little sister and that she was doing this for my own good. That I had let her down and that I was a stupid girl. Because of the cuts and bruises to my body I didn't go to school for a week. I never failed another exam ever."

There is a powerful technique to manage trauma such as this and over our subsequent sessions I used it repeatedly with Mae.

I invited Mae to sit in a chair facing away from me. I asked Mae to talk out loud to the chair opposite in which sat an imaginary thirteen-year-old little Mae. I asked adult Mae to talk to little Mae. I sat behind her and where appropriate I prompted her. I started by getting Mae to say in an adult voice, "Little Mae, what happened to you that day was wrong. It was not your fault. I know that you were terrified. I know that you were cruelly treated and I am here for you. I know that mum was very wrong to do what she did. Indeed, she committed a criminal act in abusing you. Whatever happens in the future to you, little Mae, I will be here for you. I will protect you from this type of abuse ever happening to you again. I love you and what happened to you that day was wrong. I know, little Mae, that you are not stupid and that you were abused by mum. It won't happen again."

Over the next five or six session we repeated this process. As Mae got more familiar with the process, she became more angry about her mother's treatment of little Mae. Mae became more realistic about the control that her mother had over her life. In a critical moment Mae realised that her mother had worked so hard on their education to fulfil her own needs; to be able to brag to neighbours, friends, colleagues and relatives about how clever and successful her children were.

On our last session, some six months after her referral, Mae said, "The exam is coming up in three weeks. I think I will do okay, but if I don't pass, I will do it again next year."

I ran a line by her. I said, "Remember Mae 'parents owe children everything, children owe parents nothing.' Do the exam for yourself, not her."

Mae laughed and protested. "You're trying to make me into a banana!"

I was nonplussed. "Sorry," I said, "what do you mean?"

"Ha," said Mae "you are western, you don't understand, in my culture we owe our parents for our lives. You can't make me yellow on the outside and white on the inside like a banana."

I laughed, "Well, I guess I had to try, didn't I?"

She smiled and said, "I'll let you know about the exam."

Some three months later I got a postcard from Singapore. On the back was written, "I failed."

A year later I got another post card from Singapore. On the back was written, "I passed."

Some six months later, I got a referral to see a teenage boy who had been traumatised by seeing his dad killed in a road traffic accident in which he was also injured. It was signed by a doctor I didn't know.

I would have missed the connection but in ballpoint at the bottom of the letter was written aka Dr. Mae Liu, Consultant Paediatrician.

I was pleased. I am also sure that her mother would have been proud. I also have no doubt that she would have seen her daughter's success as validation of her appalling parenting.

Chapter Fifteen

"I'd slap the little cunt"

Jodi attended the group for the first time. For adults, with the usual neglect and abusive childhood backgrounds coming into the unknown can be very challenging. Is the environment safe? Can I trust people? Can I get a seat by the door? Can I escape if I have to? Is a man running the group? Am I safe?

Within minutes of group starting, I was aware Jodi was becoming agitated. Her left foot was tapping the ground, her shoulders were hunched and her body was taut. She was scanning the group, her eyes flickering around the room. Without drawing direct attention to her distress (she was not the only hypervigilant, over-aroused person in the room), I invited the group to do some breathing. "Ocean breathing is good. Imagine you are standing by the ocean. Breathe in through your nose, out through your mouth, take your time, but keep your breathing going in a circle, keep the flow going."

A routine breathing exercise that for most group members was soothing. I watched carefully. The old hands had their eyes closed and were taking slow rhythmic breaths. Not Jodi; her eyes were wide open, her breathing shallow and rapid. Before I could intervene she stood up and said, "What the fuck is this?" The group leapt to a halt, all eyes open, some wary, some critical, some compassionate.

For some traumatised adults, inviting them to close their eyes and breathe is the worst possible thing to ask of them because in shutting your eyes, you can become vulnerable to attack.

I said, "Sorry, Jodi, my mistake, coming into a group of strangers and there I was trying to get you to close your eyes. When you feel like you do now, what do you need?"

Jodi was on it, "I need to feel safe."

"How can we help you do that?"

Jodi said, "I need to know everybody's name and what they are doing here and I need him to leave." With that, she pointed to Phil, a wiry, cadaverous, mild-mannered man with a history of severe childhood neglect that he had masked with years of drinking.

When such things happen in group it's always a difficult call. Do you sacrifice one patient because of the demands of another? However, my preference was always to explore. What was it about Phil that was so challenging? What threat did he pose?

However, Phil was an old hand and he beat me to it.

"Jodi," he said, "who do I remind you of?"

Jodi said, "My father who raped me."

Phil stood up and said, "I'm sorry," and with great dignity, left the room.

There is a benefit to understanding that the overwhelming majority, if not all, adults who attend an inpatient or day patient unit, are there because of childhood neglect and abuse. The benefit is that you can "train up" not only the staff, but also the other group members, to better manage traumatised patients. In so doing, they also come to understand themselves better. Later with Phil, I thanked him for his compassion and generosity in leaving, and also teased him that he appeared to have more compassion for a stranger than for himself.

On Phil's departure, Jodi calmed. I used Jodi's need for safety to both get everyone to introduce themselves, say why they had attended group, and also recall what it had been like coming to their first session.

An hour passed, we broke for morning tea and I reflected that Jodi, although clearly threatened by being in a group, had also been assertive (angry) enough to state that she wanted Phil to leave.

When group recommenced I said, "Jodi, I wonder if you'd be prepared to do an exercise that may be challenging?"

Jodi nodded abruptly.

I turned toward Jodi and said, "I want you to imagine that you are walking alongside a river. You are following a path. It's a warm, pleasant day and the path takes you toward a large, open park space. As you follow the path you see in the distance some playground equipment, which, of course, is unremarkable. However, as you follow the path further it takes you toward the playground and you observe that someone is playing on one of the swings. Again this is unremarkable, but as you walk right by the swings you become aware that there is a little six or seven-year-old girl, slowly swinging on one of the swings. She is all alone, there is no one else nearby. She is quietly crying. What would you do?"

Jodi paused and said, "I really don't know."

I waited, the group waited, and then Jodi slowly repeated, "I really don't know," and then a little later, "I think I would just carrying on walking."

My experience from using this exercise with lots of patients told me that this was an unusual answer. After all, in similar circumstances, what would you do?

The usual answer is to at least offer some help and assistance. What is interesting, is that if you present this scenario to adults who have had good childhoods, they always say something like, "oh, I'd sit on the swing next to her and tell her that I was there for her and would stay with her until she was calm and safe." They know what to do because when they were young, it was done for them. Jodi's answer clearly indicated that such nurturing had not occurred for her.

The value of this exercise though lies in its repetition, with a twist.

So I said to Jodi, "I want you to imagine, just like before, that you are walking along by a river and exactly as before the path takes you toward a park and you see some playground equipment and as you get closer, just like before, you notice that someone is slowly swinging on one of the swings. However, unlike before, this time when you pass by the swings you see that there is a little six-year-old girl on the swings and that little girl is you. What would you do?"

Without hesitation, without a pause, Jodi said, "I'd slap the little cunt."

The group gasped.

I said, "Because?"

"Because she's pathetic," said Jodi.

"Because?"

"Because she needs to toughen up and get on with it."

"Because?"

"Because," said Jodi, "otherwise she will die."

I said, "I understand." And I did.

I understood because my father had spent his childhood in an orphanage and had no time for "nonsense." He knew that in order to survive in an orphanage, you needed to be tough, to be self-reliant, to never be vulnerable, never look weak, never sit on a swing and cry. You had to get on and be tough.

I also understood because most of my patients were determined never to give themselves an inch.

So I said to Jodi, "What did six-year-old you have to manage and get on with?"

"Having sex with dad, being physically abused by mum, being bullied by my brothers and never having a friend."

Later writing up her notes, I saw that she had five diagnoses, namely borderline personality disorder, major depression, alcohol dependence, bipolar disorder, and generalised anxiety disorder.

Although Jodi's response was very harsh, my guess is that it was lifesaving. If as a six-year-old you become overwhelmed by what is being done to you, become overwhelmed by the neglect and the abuse, realise that there is no way out and that you cannot cope, then the solution is suicide. Every year, children as young as five kill themselves because they realise that the people who were supposed to nurture them are neglecting them and abusing them. Suicide is a leading cause of death in young people aged five to seventeen.

Adopting a tough, don't-be-so-pathetic stance may keep you alive long enough to come to terms with what happened to you.

Jodi was forty-nine. Over the following four years, Jodi was re-admitted five times to detox from her use of alcohol and other drugs. She participated in day patient group care and hours of psychotherapy to get her to where she is today; a grandmother, a teacher's assistant and someone who likes herself.

About a year ago Jodi, after an absence of some two years, popped into the S & T group. Coincidentally, Phil was there that day. They hugged each other.

As the group progressed, Phil took an opportunity and asked Jodi how she was. Jodi then told of the exercise that she had done some five or six years earlier. She told of how she didn't know what to do with a little lost stranger, but knew exactly what to do with her own vulnerable self. She repeated her words exactly, "I'd slap the little cunt."

She then said, "But now I know what to do with the little lost girl. I'd sit on the swing beside her. I'd tell her I was there for her. I'd tell her that I too knew what it was like to be all alone and afraid. I wouldn't leave her until she was sorted."

"As for me," she continued, "I'd pick her up give her a hug, tell her I'd always be there for her and that I loved her."

With that she went to the large shopping bag she always had with her, rummaged around and pulled out a battered rag doll.

She said to the group, "For the past five years we haven't gone anywhere without each other. This is little six-year-old me. Bill made me buy her, to make me softer toward myself, more compassionate toward little me."

She sat in group that day being charming and smiling and helpful and considerate to others, holding her rag doll.

The one that I absolutely never told her to buy.

Chapter Sixteen

The apple of his mother's eye

Every now and then a patient will answer a question with an answer so astounding, so surprising, that instantly they become understandable. Suddenly the morass they are in makes total sense.
Geoffrey was one such patient. The initial referral was far from encouraging.

Dear Bill,
Please will you see Geoffrey Chambers. He is a middle-aged man who has long-term, treatment-resistant, depression. He has run the gamut of antidepressants, ECT and TMS without any significant improvement. He has, and I have to say somewhat reluctantly, agreed to give psychotherapy a try. Please see and advise.
Good luck!
Regards Dr. N G

On first sight, Geoffrey looked older than his fifty-one years. He walked in to my office with an air of resigned defeat. If anyone ever carried their own personal rain cloud, it was Geoffrey. When I asked my standard "what brings you to see a psychologist?" question, he wearily replied, "My psychiatrist told me I had to come and see you, I've been depressed for as long as I can remember."

Depression is very interesting. Although the psychiatric text books will outline depression in a standard, "these are the symptoms of depression" manner, the truth is that depression "is highly individually coloured." In effect, everyone's depression is different.

So I asked Geoffrey, "What is your type of depression like?"

He pondered his answer. And then slowly said, "It's heavy, it's monotonous, it's weary, it's never ending, it's impossible. I've been depressed since I was young and nothing makes any difference."

He stopped and then looked up at me. "Look no offence, but I don't think talking to you is going to make any difference either. I've tried psychotherapy before and it didn't work." The room was filled with his defeat.

My immediate reaction was to counter his pessimism and say how effective talking therapy is. However, I managed to catch myself entering that reassurance dead-end trap and I took a moment and reflected on how *I* was feeling. I was feeling powerless, defeated, but also angry.

I realised I was feeling him. So I countered with, "How angry are you feeling?"

He looked up at me surprised. He said with energy, "Very."

"Because?"

"Because it's not fair, I didn't ask to be depressed, I didn't want to be useless and hopeless and lonely. I've tried all my life to be good and yet here I am. It's just not fair."

"Tell me about being good?"

He went back into himself. I could almost see him shrink.

"My mum and dad were very loving, but very strict, especially my dad. I knew that I needed to be what they wanted, be a good boy and toe the line. All my life I've done what they wanted and after dad died, about ten years ago, I now do what mum wants."

I countered again, "And the anger?"

"What makes me rage is that my younger brother never did what they wanted. He just did what he wanted and still does and he still gets away with it!"

"Can you give me an example of his 'getting away with it'?"

Geoffrey paused. "Yes," he said, "our bikes."

"Bikes?"

"When I was ten and he was eight, we were given bikes for Christmas. My dad was very clear that the bikes were expensive and we needed to look after them. I kept my bike in tip-top condition. I looked after it, was careful when I used it, and after a couple of years it still looked like new. Yet, my brother just hooned around on his; it was always dirty and scratched and he frequently had punctures and other problems and he didn't give a shit. After two years, his bike was a wreck and he got a new one. When I protested dad just said I didn't need a new one because mine 'looked like new.'"

"So," I said, "bring me up to date, how does being good look now?"

He pursed his lips and in a low small voice said, "I've sort of given up being good. I'm sort of passive. I just try not to upset anyone."

A reminder from Dorothy Rowe – "Depression is a prison where you are both the suffering prisoner and the cruel jailer."

"How powerless do you feel? How defeated?"

"Totally," he said. "I'm just stuck in a mire."

WHAT HAPPENED?

"Tell me about that mire?"

Geoffrey looked at the floor. His posture reeked defeat and hopelessness.

He emotionlessly said, "Every day is the same. I live at my brother's place. It's an old home near the beach he's going to knock down and build his dream home on. But, until he does, he lets me live there rent-free. It's really appalling, there's no heating or air con, and when it rains it leaks, but as he says there's no point in fixing anything because it's going to be bulldozed. I also look after his dog; she's an old kelpie. I get up every morning and take her for a walk along the beach. Then I usually go to my mum's. Since dad died, mum is quite lonely, so every day I go over to her house for lunch. She lives in South Perth, the house is beautiful, right on the river.

"It's funny, but she lent me dad's old car. I've had it since he died. It's a very old rusty Ford Falcon. It's a wreck, looks shit; so mum won't let me park it in her drive, I have to park it in the car park opposite!"

I am taken by his lack of having anything of his own. He had a borrowed house, car and dog, and an enervating sense of being at the behest of others.

I continued to explore his typical day.

"How are your lunches with mum?"

"Pretty dreadful, she usually cajoles me about my life, tells me how well Ben, my brother the successful property developer, is doing and how much she enjoys catching up with his wife Marie, and seeing the grandchildren."

The making of odious comparisons, whether done by others or by oneself, is a common companion in depression.

Geoffrey paused for a minute. I wondered if he was putting things together, his beholdenness, his lack of personal agency, the transient nature of his existence.

However, he wasn't.

He said, "I don't know what I'd do without my mum and brother. I'd be all on my own, no home, no car, no support." He sank into sadness, inadequacy and self-loathing.

I said, "How long have you been living like this?"

"Oh," he said, "for as long as I remember. I've always lived with my brother or in one of his derelict houses. I've had lunch with mum every day for the past thirty years and I've never worked or owned my own car or anything."

I was suddenly struck by something, how did Geoffrey survive financially?

So I asked, "Geoffrey, how do you support yourself, are you on a disability pension?"

Geoffrey quickly, tetchily countered, "Oh I'm not that bad. My mum gives me an allowance each week. It's not much but it keeps me going."

Beholden even more, trapped even more.

The session ended. I made him an appointment for the following week and I said genuinely that I had enjoyed meeting him and talking to him. He replied "Thank you," then added, "I don't feel any better."

Geoffrey opened his next appointment by noting that nothing had changed. He had, in the previous week, visited his mother every day for lunch. His biggest concern was that the refrigerator in his brother's house had "died" and this meant that he now needed to buy small cartons of milk every day. He was not sure if he could afford to replace the refrigerator.

I asked him how he felt about his reliance on his mum for money. He corrected me and said that the money his mother gave him each week (about five hundred dollars), was actually drawn from his bank account and his mother just managed his money, as she had always done.

I was curious about this fund. Given that he reported that he had never worked or had social security benefits, where had it come from?

Geoffrey recalled his mother had told him that she had always wanted to have children, but doubted whether she could because of a childhood illness. Thus, she had told Geoffrey that when she discovered she was pregnant, she was delighted. From the moment of the confirmation of the pregnancy, his mother had put ten dollars a day into what she called, "The Geoffrey Fund." (He was named after his mother's brother who had drowned when aged seven). His mother told Geoffrey that from the moment he was born, and as a child "he was the apple of her eye."

As a small child, Geoffrey and his mother would go to the local bank every Friday and put seventy dollars in cash into The Geoffrey Fund. He said she still did it to this very day, although now the Friday transaction was done electronically.

Geoffrey noted that after his brother was born, he realised Ben did not get the same treatment. Geoffrey admitted that he was secretly pleased that his brother did not get the weekly dividend.

Geoffrey continued to talk about how as a young child he felt very special and delighted in being "the apple of his mother's eye." In order to maintain this accolade, he said he knew he had to be very good and he was careful not to upset his mum in any way. He noted that his mother would sometimes confide that she found his brother difficult on occasions, and she was very pleased that the apple of her eye was such a good boy.

I asked Geoffrey to reflect on the paralysis in his life and the apparent success of the "less good" Ben. He said he couldn't explain it. Ben was, he reflected, "always his own person," whereas Geoffrey never was.

I invited him to reflect on his beholdenness, that maybe being the apple of someone's eye was a very hard act to maintain. He, however, refuted this and posited, "Where would I be without mum?" I tried at various times to infer that maybe, just maybe, he needed to "divorce" his mother and escape to freedom. Geoffrey reiterated his dependence upon her, how good she was and if it wasn't for her and his brother he would be homeless, probably dead.

Over the next few sessions we attempted other ways of understanding why Geoffrey was so stuck. But, to no avail. Both of us realised we were getting stuck, going over the same ground. It was frustrating and I noted to Geoffrey that the sessions seemed to reflect his life. He agreed and with a strong tinge of hopelessness said, "I knew psychotherapy was not going to work."

In Australia at that time, everyone (with a GP referral) was entitled each year to six sessions of psychotherapy that were partially funded by the Federal Government. Geoffrey noted that as we had done five of them, he would attend for the sixth session, but he would terminate his therapy because he "obviously couldn't afford to pay the going rate" without the government subsidy.

At the end of the session, I wondered to him whether The Geoffrey Fund might be able to subsidise his on-going therapy. I casually asked him how much was in the fund, and Geoffrey replied that he didn't know, he'd have to ask mum. He said he'd never been brave enough to ask, but that, if I insisted, he would ask. I said, "Well, you do need a new fridge … and more therapy."

I wondered, given the paralysis of the last session and his sense of psychotherapy not working, whether he would attend for his potentially last appointment. I was pleased when he did.

I asked the usual "how's your world?" question and Geoffrey replied, "Confusing, interesting, surprising." He said it with a degree of energy.

This surprised me, so I said, "Because?"

"Because there is $3.2 million in The Geoffrey Fund."

I could not contain my astonishment. "What, how did that happen?"

"My mum is very good with money. Apparently from the time I was eighteen, she invested the money in different shares and with all the dividends just bought more shares. Over the years it has accumulated."

He paused and said, "I told her I wanted some money to see you and buy a new fridge. She said Okay to you, but I could only buy a second-hand fridge."

I looked at Geoffrey and said, "Help me understand. You are a millionaire yet you are asking mum for permission to buy a fridge?"

Geoffrey paused and said, "After mum told me I was worth three million dollars I was so confused that I walked straight out of her house and for the next two hours walked around the river. I remembered something. I know why I am as I am."

Geoffrey looked at me, and said with tears in his eyes, "I was seven years old and I was with mum and Ben in the local newsagent's. Mum had always said that The Geoffrey Fund was my money, was 'apple of my eye money.' It was a Friday, we had earlier gone to the bank and put the seventy dollars into The Geoffrey Fund so I was aware that I had 'money.' I was browsing through the shelves of magazines while my mother and Ben were buying some crayons. I saw some comics and started to read one. I became enthralled by one cartoon story and picked the comic up and ran to mum and said, 'Hey mum can I have some money from The Geoffrey Fund to buy this comic, it's really good.'"

Geoffrey paused; he was literally, shaking silently. I coaxed him "What happened?"

Geoffrey said, in a soft, young, voice, "My mother slapped me very hard across the face and screamed at me. She said, 'I have saved that money for you for your future. It's not to be wasted on rubbish like comics. Comics are a trick because next week you will want to buy the next one and then where will you be? You want to squander away your future. I won't allow it. I have never been so disappointed in you. I will not have you being so careless with money. Money is important, it must never, never be wasted.'"

Geoffrey said that his mother then snatched the comic out of his hand and marched him home where he was told to go to his room and not come out until he had learned the value of money.

I looked at Geoffrey, he was crying. "You must have felt totally shamed."

Geoffrey said that he was mortified that he had let his mother down so much. He said that there and then he decided that his money was somehow not really his, and that he would never ask his mother for "his" money again. He said that he relied on her throughout his life to know best about his money and how to manage it properly. He said he never wanted to ask for money ever again.

When he returned a week later, Geoffrey was different. He was taller.

The "How's your world?" question was succinctly answered.

He replied, "I think it's time I looked after myself."

"Because?"

He said, "Because being the apple of someone's eye is a terrible responsibility. I need to disappoint her."

He got no argument from me.

It took Geoffrey two months to buy a new fridge, six months to buy a new (second-hand) car and a year to buy a house. When I last heard of him, he also had a girlfriend.

I just hope he wasn't the apple of her eye.

Chapter Seventeen

Running on empty

Psychotherapy is a process not an event. The general rule of thumb is that the longer people engage in psychotherapy the better they do. Notwithstanding this, people can make very good gains within six to ten sessions. Matthew was a case in point.

His GP referred him for the management of his anxiety disorder. However, it transpired very quickly that Matthew's "anxiety" was directly related to his way of being in the world. When I asked the opening, "What brings you to see a psychologist?" question, Mathew replied by saying "I'm stuck. I'm not getting anywhere, in fact I'm going backwards."

"Going backwards?"

"Yes, in all sorts of ways; definitely financially, but also in my relationships with my family, with my daughter, at work and in life in general. I'm tired all the time and I'm just not getting things done."

"It sounds like you've sort of run out of steam?"

Encapsulating people's dilemmas in a metaphor can be very useful. Even if you don't get it exactly right, but are sort of in the ball park, it will work. People appreciate being understood.

Matthew quickly responded, "Yes that's it, I'm that Jackson Browne song 'Running on Empty.'"

When people say unusual things it is always worth exploring.

"Any lyrics from that song that stand out for you?"

He thought for a moment, shut his eyes and sang to himself. Then he said, "I guess I just don't know what I'm hoping to find."

He opened his eyes and looked at me. He smiled and questioned, "Got a cure for that, doc?"

I laughed. "Well, let's see shall we, tell me about running on empty?"

Matthew had just adroitly given me a very useful signpost of where to go. People who "run on empty" are giving themselves away: too much energy, both physical and psychological going out, and not enough restoration coming in. However, the question is, of course, "why be like that?"

Matthew talked about his life. His fiftieth birthday was in three weeks. He had been divorced for two years, and although he described the divorce as amicable, it had, he reported, badly impacted on his relationship with his sixteen-year-old daughter. This was largely because his jobs, working as a care assistant in a home for disabled young people and also driving his own twenty seater bus on tourist trips to the beaches and vineyards some three hours to the south, meant that he was often not available when his daughter was free. He also noted that he had a third business making kitchen cabinets. Trained as a carpenter, he had largely given carpentry away, but he noted he still made cabinets for friends and family as a sideline.

The trick of the first session with any client is to establish a rapport and engage sufficiently well to make them want to return.

Thus, in any session there is a need to tailor one's therapeutic approach to the client. My first impression of Mathew was that he was a very practical man who had a no-nonsense demeanour, coupled with a wry sense of humour.

I sensed I needed at first to be more practical and efficient than psychodynamic. Pragmatic rather than too psychological, so I asked him to complete a simple exercise, the energy egg exercise described in Chapter six.

"Matthew," I said, "on this piece of paper I'm going to draw four circles. Now Mathew you have in any week twelve 'energy eggs.' These eggs are not just about your physical energy or time but also the amount of psychological energy you put into any week. Now, how many of your energy eggs go into work?"

He looked at me with a wry look on his face. "Can I say six?" he said.

I said, "Of course, if you think that is a fair reflection of the amount of psychological and physical energy you put into work on an average week."

He smiled and very reluctantly wrote ten in the first circle. He had anticipated where we were going.

"Now," I said, "the second circle is 'home.' This includes things like paying the bills, fixing the house up, but also includes seeing members of your family of origin, seeing you daughter and catching up with friends. Everything that is part of your 'domestic existence.'"

In this circle he wrote six.

"Now," I said, "circle three is energy given to any intimate significant relationship."

He quickly wrote zero.

"And finally, the last circle is 'time for self.' These are the things you do on your own that are enjoyable, like exercising, reading, perhaps engaging in a hobby, etc."

He wrote zero.

I held out the sheet to him, "How does that look Matthew?"

He got it instantly. "Looks like I'm running on empty."

"Yes, Matthew in a twelve-energy-egg week you expend sixteen eggs on others and you have zero eggs that are restorative like time for self or having an intimate relationship. How long do you think you can keep this up?"

He smiled, "Not much longer, I'm exhausted."

The session was ending. I left him with a question to consider. "Matthew, why are you like this?"

When Matthew returned the following week he was overtly subdued. After five or so minutes of our session I noted this back to him. "Matthew, as compared to the last session, you seem to be subdued and a bit flat?"

He nodded his agreement. He said that the week had been difficult; his daughter had intimated that she did not want to see him anymore. He had worked extra shifts at his care assistant job and to top things off on a trip with tourists to the wineries, his bus had developed a serious engine problem that not only terminated the trip, but made him late back for a visit with his daughter. Matthew also reported that he could not afford to fix his bus.

"I just can't get anything right," he said.

"I'm sure it feels that way, but may I ask a question?"

"Yes."

"Why did you take extra shifts at the care centre?"

"Oh," said Matthew, "someone was ill, and the manager asked me to cover two extra shifts."

"Did you want to do those shifts?"

"No not at all, but I didn't want to let the manager down."

"Tell me about letting people down?"

Matthew went quiet. "I have been thinking about your question and why I'm always running on empty. I think I've done it all my life."

"Yes, I'm sure you have. Why do you think that is so?"

"It was how we were brought up. Dad was a volunteer emergency services worker, mum did lots for the church. We were all encouraged to give back to the community. Mum hated people being selfish. She could spot selfishness at a thousand metres and would jump on it. We only got pocket money if we had done a good deed. I used to look after the garden of our next door neighbour who had had a stroke."

He thought for a moment and said, "We always had strays in our house."

"Strays?"

"Yes, stray cats, dogs, people. I hated it. It always meant more work for me and my brothers or worse, often we had to give up our beds for other people."

"And, if you protested?"

Matthew stiffened. "Protests were dismissed out of hand. Mum would say what if Jesus couldn't have been bothered to feed the five thousand, what if the good Samaritan had walked on by? What if I decided it was too much bother to go shopping? In this house we do things for others, especially those who need our help."

We looked at each other. I said, "It's difficult to resist that message, isn't it?"

"Impossible," said Matthew. He paused, "I was named after the disciple Matthew. He was a tax collector who repented his ways and gave back to the community more than he had taken. I have to give more than I take."

"Because?"

"Because otherwise you are selfish, wicked, wrong."

"And how is your self-sacrificing working for you?"

Matthew looked up and said, "It's killing me."

I took a gamble and said, "Okay for the next week, until we meet again, I want you to go out into the world and say to yourself 'it's ME first, fuck the rest.'"

Matthew looked at me aghast. "I couldn't, I can't, I won't."

"Just bear with me, Matthew. How would it be if you did, just for a week, put yourself first?"

He sat up straight, he interlocked his fingers and then sat completely still. Then, looking straight through me, he said, "It would be wonderful."

Although there were still some five or so minutes of the session remaining he stood up said, "Thank you," and left.

I was very pleased when he attended his next appointment as I was worried I had been too confronting, too direct.

I asked him, "How's your week been?"

"Different, difficult, painful, rewarding, freeing and surprising."

"Tell me."

He told me that immediately after he had seen me he had to go and give a quote on making some kitchen cabinets, for a friend of a friend. He did not want to do the job, he was too busy, it would be a chore but he felt that he should do it. He ought to do it. He said, "Bill, as you can imagine they were common feelings, but I was somehow very aware of them."

Matthew noted that as he travelled there, he decided on a plan as to how he could get out of the job, but without appearing to say no. He would merely charge them double his usual price.

I stopped him and said, "Um, my 'ME first fuck the rest' perspective probably means that you should have phoned them and told them to find someone else!"

Matthew laughed, "Well, I'm not so sure you're right!"

"Oh, okay, so what happened?"

Matthew said that when he entered the house, the wife made him very welcome, made him a coffee and showed him exactly what she wanted. He said it was a relatively straight-forward job. Matthew said the client wanted the cabinets made from materials he already had in stock so it would be quick and easy to make the cabinets at his home workshop and then bring them to the house to install them. Matthew said the "old Matthew" kicked in and he estimated the cost of the job, at mate's rates, to be seven thousand dollars. He knew that the price was very good for them; he was literally doing them a favour.

Matthew then stopped talking. I prompted, "Go on what happened?"

He said, "Just as I was going to say to her seven thousand dollars I realised that I didn't want the work, it would take up time I could spend with my daughter and get in the way of any 'me time' I might conjure up. So I thought, 'I'll just double the quote.' As I was writing the quote out I got so nervous, I was literally sweating, I was going against everything I had been taught, I was not helping her, but I doubled the price anyway and handed her the sheet with the new 'please reject it' quote on it."

I was enthralled, "Okay what happened?"

He laughed, "She accepted my quote on the spot!"

I was just about to remonstrate with him and tell him that ME first means saying no directly, that subterfuges don't work, but something in his manner stopped me.

"Bill," he said, "in my anxiety I got the arithmetic wrong, I'd quoted her sixteen thousand dollars. I've told my daughter we are going to Bali on holiday.

"Do you know Bill, I think I've under-priced myself all my life, I've not valued myself enough. And you'll be really pleased with me, I refused to do two extra shifts at work and I'm also going to increase the amount I charge for the trips down south."

I looked at him. He smiled and said, "I may be overdoing it but I've joined a dating site. I got my daughter to help with my profile. We titled it, 'I know what I'm hoping to find.'"

Chapter Eighteen

Some reflections on being a psychotherapist

Being a psychotherapist is a tough gig, particularly if you take a trauma-informed perspective. Often you will hear things that, although they no longer surprise, they will disturb. You will hear of child neglect, of incest, of unspeakable cruelty, of rape. You will hear about violence, controlled and uncontrolled. You will hear of murder. You will be told of atrocities. You will have patients who kill themselves. There are stories of corrupt police officers, dodgy doctors and swindling siblings. You'll hear of grandfathers who sell their granddaughters to their paedophilic mates. You will despair for humankind.

You will also hear a plethora of what, in comparison, appear misdemeanours; affairs, greed, deception, theft, being stuck, being obligated, being left, being jealous, being dependent, being anxious, being psychotic. These are all still real forms of human misery.

One of the best psychotherapists I know, very experienced, very skilled, sometimes phones me on his way to work on a Monday and says, "Here I go again; there is already a wisp of mustard gas wafting into the trenches."

It doesn't matter how experienced you are, how good your therapeutic alliances are, how honourable your work. Every day is a challenge. Every day you may get caught out. You may fall short. The argument you had with your spouse may intrude, the finances may feel an impossible burden and then there's a colleague complaining about the practice manager's time-keeping.

You find yourself shutting off. The intensity of six, seven, eight, nine sessions in a day means that as you drive home, the idea of dealing with dinner, the dog, the daughters, the partner and life in general, holds little appeal. After a day of rape, murder and mayhem, squabbles over homework, who's cooking or what the neighbour said, pale into the infinitesimal.

Similarly, those dinner parties or social events, being polite, engaging in small talk, the latest Donald Trump escapades, troubles with the decorator, the cost of avocados, or heaven forbid, why Freda's Aunt Jane said what she did, are all likely to invoke ennui of unbearable depth. Every now and then, a topic at a dinner party will come up and your treatise on why, for example, Cardinal George Pell can be both a "good man" and a rapist, will invoke outrage in the listeners, but comments by the also attending airline pilot about turbulence over the equator will be met with awed reverence. Why does everyone think they are an expert on being human?

So, how to survive this tsunami of human pain? Dr. Anthony Storr in his book *Solitude* wrote about the importance of solitude for psychotherapists.

Based on what I read, here is my take on what the optimum lifestyle for a psychotherapist is:

Essentially the life of the psychotherapist needs to be solitudinous one; arguably to live alone in a serviced apartment. Thus, you could wake early and go for a jog in an adjacent park before eating a modest breakfast. You then walk contemplatively through the park to your office. Over the years you will get to into the rhythm of the park and its seasons. This slow ebb and flow of light, of growth, of temperature will be soothing; the ever-ness of time.

On arriving in good time at the office you carefully read the case notes, pulled out by the secretary, of the four persons you will see that that morning.

Having seen those four patients, you then walk to the park and eat the lunch you collect from a nearby deli. On autumn and winter days you enjoy soup and a roll, in summer, a salad. The British spring is unpredictable so usually soup, but on some days that promise summer, a salad. Your lunch always awaits your collection. As you pick up your lunch you nod, but never speak, to the deli's owner. The bill is paid monthly by your secretary, out of practice funds, a tax deductible item. You eat your lunch alone, either in the park, or when raining, in the library in your office.

After lunch you return to the office, you peruse the case notes of the four people you have scheduled for the afternoon. At six o'clock you allow yourself a half hour to complete your notes and return any phone calls. You may on the way home, phone a psychotherapist colleague for no other reason than to "just chat."

On arriving home you shower and then eat the dinner that has been laid out for you by the cleaner/maid/cook who services your, and two others', apartments in the same block.

After dinner you have time for reading, reflection, playing music or, in carefully limited doses, an episode of a police drama. You go to bed. You get up in the morning and do it all over again.

At the weekends you arise earlier and go running with a psychotherapist colleague. After an hour or so of running you stop for coffee and a croissant with your colleague. You reflect on any patient irritations or issues that have arisen during the week. After coffee you return home. You do chores, you clean, you organise. You impose order on a disordered world.

You may in the afternoon visit an art exhibition or play bridge at the local club where they think you are a businessman. On Sundays you repeat the morning run, but may drive to and then walk on a local rural pathway. Twice a month you have sex with the maid/cleaner, but she never stays over.

After I wrote this and re-read it, I felt very soothed.

Ah, if only. I showed it to my wife (who is also a psychotherapist). She read it, she hesitated and said perspicaciously, "Well, doesn't that that just reflect your childhood and what you've told me about Dr. Storr and his own isolated childhood."

"I think," she continued, "that we all need to understand our default position when it comes to psychological distress."

She paused, "Don't you use that 'eight-year-old kid going home distressed and what do you do next' exercise?"

"Yes," I said, "I really like that exercise, it's always very telling."

"Um," she said, "I think you're just lusting for your old ways of being and managing your distress with splendid isolation, you know, you go for protection, but," (sounding very pleased with herself), "don't you always insist that your patients manage their distress my making bids for connection? Soothe by leaning into their relationships."

She was on a roll, "Didn't you last week lecture that being vulnerable is the key to coping? That vulnerability is a strength and invincibility a weakness? That being vulnerable is the key to compassion and self-soothing?"

She was annoyingly right and I thought about how, over the years, I had managed the burden of being a psychotherapist. Once again, my wife was right. I had soothed by connection. It's the only way to go.

I realised that I had developed my own remedy (as we must all do) for that perennial wafting mustard gas. I have realised a number of things that I share here for consideration.

First, I have no one in my personal life who does not add to it. All my friends and acquaintances have to value-add to my life; now there is connection. Any psychological drains are ruthlessly dispatched to the "used to be friends" gulag.

Two, for the past twenty years, I have had a mate (also a psychotherapist) who runs with me. Every Saturday, most Sundays, rain hail or shine, we run together, we talk, we connect, we soothe each other. Once, we even ran a marathon together, and although at thirty-two kilometres he left me behind, I later had the delightful triumph of being served the last remaining magnificent steak au poivre available in a late night Parisienne bistro.

Three, if I go out for dinner, it is usually with only one other person. That way I can have a reasonably meaningful conversation (more connection).

Four, and most importantly, the trick of the psychotherapist's life, is to have a partner who is able to travel with you through your life as a therapist. As noted above, my wife is also a psychotherapist. Sometimes when we get home at the end of the day, the best we can do is to walk the dog, eat dinner and then sit together watching TV in restorative, companionable silence.

Oh, and five. I am very clear with my patients that I work for three months and then have a month off. In that month off I have nothing to do with psychologists, psychology or anything remotely connected to work. My wife and I re-connect, we travel. I walk long distances with a friend, run, and I eat and drink too much. I sometimes travel with my daughters. I only socialise with a few close friends, who never, well, hardly ever, talk about their lives.

As a psychotherapist you will see six, seven, eight, nine, sometimes perhaps even ten patients in a day. With each, you will make an individual, intimate connection. You will be honoured with their trust. There will be moments of great vulnerability, realisations, "aha" moments, and insight. You will play mind detectives together and discover new truths. *They will tell you things they have never told anyone.* You will feel shame turn to self-compassion, self-loathing into self-acceptance. You will see psychosis evaporate. You will have clear evidence of lives changed for the better. You will may even save a life and thereby, save the world. You will also hear stories that make you marvel at human compassion, and the capacity of people to move beyond the shackles of their pasts. There will be stories of courage and the confrontation of demons. You will marvel at the human spirit and the capacity to repair even the most harrowing of childhoods, and you will know deep inside that you have played a part.

Being a psychotherapist really is the best job in town.

Chapter Nineteen
Conclusion

I am writing this concluding chapter after a day of being a psychotherapist. I saw six patients. I had in their referral letters been informed that the first client had an "anti-social personality disorder." The second was "depressed," and the third was a woman with a "generalised anxiety disorder." The fourth had almost been killed at work and then, while recuperating, almost killed by a passing motorist; a case of PTSD. The fifth had an "adjustment disorder" and the sixth, "alcohol dependence."

Yet, what I heard was respectively was (1) "my childhood was fucked," (2) "I was always told I was not good enough," (3) "my uncle took advantage of me for six, maybe seven, years," (4) "I keep having nightmares about dying," (5) "my parents ran a deli, they worked from 6am until 9pm, I never understood why they had kids," and, (6) "My parents loved alcohol, arguing and hitting me."

Six ordinary, everyday patients in a psychotherapy practice; all with a variety of diagnoses, all had been offered "anti-depressants" and/or benzodiazepines. Three out of the six were relying on such psychopharmacology to cope, possibly cure, the alleged biological deficit that was causing them grief.

Yet all were, from my perspective, cases of either complex (childhood) or "simple" post-traumatic stress disorder.

So here, in a single day of work, is the critical matter that this book is about.

Do we continue with a medical model of invented diagnoses of mental illnesses of unknown biological causes, treated with drugs of dubious therapeutic capacity that alter brain chemistry and cause side effects and withdrawal syndromes? Or do we have a revolution and reject this "emperor with no clothes" paradigm and embrace a new way?

The twentieth century philosopher, Thomas Kuhn, in his book *The Structure of Scientific Revolutions,* persuasively argued that science does not, as is generally thought, develop linearly in steady increments. Kuhn demonstrated what, in fact, occurs are "paradigm shifts." In effect, scientific knowledge is only changed by conflict, by crisis, by revolution.

Kuhn argued that the process of coming to a new understanding has five stages. The first stage he labelled as "normal science." It is the uncontested acceptance of the current, dominant understanding of any particular phenomenon. However, as increasing disconfirming evidence is found and articulated, there is what Kuhn called "model drift;" a moving away from the current belief behind the explanation of the phenomenon, for example, believing the Earth is flat.

Then as even more contradictory evidence is found and the discontent with the existing model rises, a "crisis" develops. This is followed by a "revolution;" a coup de grace of the old way and the new paradigm is installed; we know the Earth is round because we have seen it from space! Peace and quiet returns and a "normal" state is achieved; well, for a while.

It would be delightful to say that the disconfirming evidence surrounding the currently dominant medical/biological/psychiatric/psychopharmacological model of mental illness is now so persuasive and so overwhelming that psychiatry is at a crisis point where revolutionaries can cause a paradigm shift.

However, as Kuhn noted, citing the Roman Catholic Church's opposition to Copernicus' challenge to the "scientific knowledge" that the earth revolved around the sun; there are always vested interests in the status quo. The dominant biological mental illness paradigm has many supporters, not least, the profession of psychiatry, general medicine and "Big Pharma." Unfortunately, it is also a *comfortable* paradigm for many persons with childhood trauma. A pill for every ill, and biological brain chemistry imbalances hold considerable passive appeal.

There have, over the past twenty years, been an increasing number of highly critical, well-argued texts that challenge the status quo. Hopefully, this book will augment that chorus of complaint. My take is that the dominant psychiatric discourse on mental health is drifting; there are increasing signs that all is not well. Can we make this drift into a crisis of discontent? Perhaps even a revolution?

This book started with the invitation to believe six impossible things. Here to finish are six very "possible to believe" quotations.

> "Who will be accountable for the many millions of individuals throughout the world taking medicines of dubious value for conditions of dubious diagnostic validity, while key figures who determine funding and shape research in psychiatric neuroscience still cling to the dream of molecular explanations and molecular interventions?"
> Prof. Nikolas Rose

"This industry has no foundation, in no way serves us and this psychiatric rule needs to end. Given that psychiatry is blatantly not the answer to life's woes, but indeed one of the causes thereof, and given that there will always be some need to for extensive emotional support what do we put in its stead?"
Dr. Bonnie Burstow

"… psychiatry, in league with the pharmaceutical industry chooses to perpetuate two fundamental hoaxes. The first is that the suffering that we call mental illness has a biological basis. The second hoax follows on from the first namely that today's drugs treatments target and correct this chemical imbalance, just like antibiotics fight infection or insulin treats diabetes …"
Luke Montagu (aka Viscount Hinchingbrooke)

"What would happen if psychiatrists told you that they don't know what illness (if any) is causing your anxiety, depression or agitation and then, if they thought it warranted, told you that there are drugs that might help, although they don't really know why or at what cost to your brain, or whether you will be able to stop taking them if you want to; nor can they guarantee that you -or your child- won't become obese of diabetic or die early and then they offer you a prescription?"
Prof. Gary Greenberg

"Pushing remedies at people instead of listening to them is a very old story. From eighteenth century bloodletting and purging, to twentieth century psychosurgery, ECT and neuroleptics, the preferred mode of in mind doctoring has been to deal with madness from a safe distance. Listening to people, taking their words seriously - instead of just trying to dose symptoms away - risks feelings of recognition and empathy."
Barbara Taylor

"Mental health problems are essentially social and psychological issues. We should replace diagnosis with straightforward descriptions of people problems [and] radically reduce the use of medications. We need to understand how each person has learned to make sense of their worlds and tailor help to their unique and complex needs."
Prof. Peter Kinderman

Please feel free to add your voice to the above discontent and ferment a crisis, or even a revolution. It is sorely needed.

Chapter Twenty

Finale

Now to finish with something a bit different.
If a patient enters an individual or group session carrying something that they don't normally bring into session, comment on it.

Claudia came back to the second half of an S & T group carrying a bunch of flowers.

She was also some fifteen minutes late; the second half was well under way. Flowers and being that late were unusual. I said to her, "Welcome back to S & T. Now what have you brought to group?"

"Ah," said Claudia, "I have bought flowers for Justine."

Justine looked up, startled. Although one of the founding members of S & T, Claudia now lived many kilometres away from the hospital and only came to the group once or twice a year. Justine was a much more recent and regular attendee. They had never, apart from that morning, ever met. Hence, Justine queried in surprise, "For me?"

"Yes," said Claudia. "Look I went to Woollies during the lunch break and as I walked past the flowers, I got a bump. Someone was saying to buy you flowers. It was an aunt of yours. She told me she had passed when you were five."

"Ah," said Justine, as though this was the most normal conversation in the world, "thanks, that's wonderful, that was my aunt Emily. You know she was the only person who ever made me feel special." Claudia handed over the flowers.

Uncertain as to the nature of what had occurred, I picked up on one aspect of the conversation. At the very beginning of my career, Anthony Thorley, a very astute British psychiatrist, once said to me, "Bill, if you don't understand something that happens in a group, always ask the patient. They will love to explain it to you and you will learn."

So, I said, "Bump?"

"Oh yes," said Claudia, "Every now and again and I get a physical push, like someone bumping into me, and it's always a sign that someone wants to talk. So, I always stop and listen. Justine's aunt told me to buy flowers."

I knew something weird was happening. I wondered if Claudia, a victim of shocking sexual abuse as a child, was having a psychotic moment.

"Oh," said Claudia, "if it's okay I'll continue … there's more."

I looked at the group. Everyone was attentive and engaged.

In for a penny …

I smiled at Claudia.

"Now, Max, your son says to not listen to your daughter, but to do what you want. It's your turn now."

Max nodded gravely. "Thank you Claudia, how is David?"

"He's good. He's relieved his pain is over, but he's worried about you. He knows his sister can be very demanding."

Max's wife of forty years had recently committed suicide. A tragic act because their son David had died a year or so earlier from a childhood genetic disorder.

Since I saw Max individually, I knew that his daughter was trying to prevent him from selling the family home, which was causing him considerable distress.

Max said, "Thank you, Claudia, that is very helpful, I had wondered what David's take on things would have been."

Every now and then, a patient will attend therapy who totally reminds you of someone else. It's uncanny and it disrupts your ability to gauge the patient.

Annie was a very recent newcomer to S & T, and a spitting image of Wednesday from the Adams family. She was very bright, with a dark sense of humour to match her appearance. She had been diagnosed as being depressed and cannabis dependent, but of course it was really childhood trauma.

"Now then, Annie," said Claudia matter-of-factly, "I'm a shit singer, but Sally wants me to sing a song for you."

Claudia started to sing the Bob Marley song, "Three Little Birds."

Annie joined in. They harmonised beautifully together.

When they stopped Annie was quietly crying.

I waited. Annie composed herself. She offered an explanation, "That was the song my sister Sally and I used to sing all the time before she died."

The group was silent. I sat with them in silence.

I'm a complete sceptic of the psychic. Yet, I had just witnessed something very unusual. I wasn't sure what to make of it. The group looked, however, to be all sitting very comfortably. Traumatised children learn to take things in their stride. They also become very good at scanning the environment for clues as to what is happening or is about to happen. I remember one patient noting, "I became very good at reading the wind." Claudia's shocking childhood may have made her very good at doing just that.

I ventured, "How are you feeling, Max?"

"Very good Bill, thanks."

I couldn't help myself. "Ah, Max," I said, "good isn't a feeling."

Everyone laughed. It was a standing joke that Max had no feelings.

He paused and smiled, "Is vindicated a feeling?"

I thought for a moment, "I think so!"

He sat back in his chair smiling.

"Justine, how are you feeling?" I said.

"Peaceful, soothed, relaxed, pleased, sad and connected."

I couldn't help it. "See Max … feelings." Max snorted.

"And Annie?"

She looked up through her tears and said, "I miss her. And I couldn't bear to think about her for so long. No matter how hard I tried, I couldn't escape the fear that she may be stuck somehow. But she's okay. She's free. That's all I needed to know."

That day we had, as usual, a psychology postgraduate student on placement in the hospital sitting in on the group. I had not met her before. I noted that she was very sternly dressed with strict black trousers and a white blouse buttoned right up to the top. Her presentation was very defended. She had said nothing in the group; had not joined in or asked any questions. She was very contained. I had the sense that she was one of those clinical psychology students with an impeccable academic and research pedigree, but little warmth or capacity to connect.

She asked, "Is it always like this in this group?" Her tone gave away that the question was not a neutral one, but a disapproving critical one. Clearly, the group had not been of the evidence-based CBT manual type she learned about in university.

I was busily formulating my response, a sort of buffer to her evident disapproval, something along the lines that S & T was a special group, with a membership of traumatised patients, so there was often a notable level of camaraderie and connection that allowed intense and intimate interactions, when Claudia beat me to it. And she was much more direct.

"Yes, girlie," she said, "it's always awesome, cos we're all awesome. Now why don't you just loosen your fucking self up and take a risk for God's sake. And you could start by unbuttoning that ridiculous blouse."

I couldn't help but agree. Even, if the language was a bit tough, the sentiment was right. Patients who have been abused as children spot inauthenticity in a flash. They know whom not to trust. The therapist who clings to rules, manuals, and how things ought to be done reveals their rigidity as the carapace of fragility. The best therapists, the so-called "Super Shrinks," have a capacity to quickly establish and maintain high quality therapeutic relationships. They come into a group prepared to get their hands dirty, willing to sail into the unknown and explore with their fellow travellers.

Facing the capricious mysteries of existence together is the only balm for human suffering.

It's the relationship that heals.

And there is a finale to this finale. It arrived as an email some six months after that unusual group. It was from Annie. She wrote: "Dear Bill, I want you to know that after THAT group I wrote this letter to my family." (Here, with her permission, it is reproduced).

"My dear family,

I felt that I had to write this down and read it to you so that I would say it just right. I have learned things in the past few days that irrevocably altered the way I see the world. You know me – I'm a huge sceptic; a science nerd; the girl who's always asking why. I believed that nothing happens for a reason and events are random; orchestrated only by the laws of nature. I felt great comfort in the notion that there is nothing after death, if only because my greatest fear was that believing in an afterlife might mean that Sally was somehow trapped here. I was wrong. I know how this will sound (crazy), and I wouldn't say this to you – and open up old wounds – if I wasn't convinced that what I've learnt is true. So here goes. I met a woman in group some months ago. She didn't know me or my story, but she came up to me and told me there was a young girl around me, with long, dark, flowing hair. My curiosity was piqued, and I asked her what she meant. She said that she speaks to dead people, relaying messages on their behalf to the living. I was fairly nonplussed at the time, and I pretty much dismissed it, given the information was so vague. After going through a few sessions with her, she learned my story, and I got to know her better. The more she described the girl, the more it sounded like Sally. A big laugh, braces, effervescent energy. Just about every time I saw her she told me something new. I didn't really believe it though. If anything, I became more sceptical over time, as I knew this woman had more information about Sally from my sharing in the group. I continued to be polite, but I was unconvinced.

The last group was different. In the morning, there was a strange energy in the room, and it was one of the more intense sessions I have experienced. Death was heavy in the air – one of the members had lost his son to illness, then his wife to suicide not long after. Other members were no strangers to suicidal thoughts … and then there was me. The woman started giving people messages – she said she had been trying to ignore them all day, but they were insistent. She told me that she has known quite a few young people who have suicided that don't quite fit; that they are brand new souls and most of them suicide because they are homesick for heaven. Somewhere in their feeling's memory their body remembers where they fit. Yes, I know how cheesy it sounds … but the way she talks about it, it's a placeholder term for the hereafter. She said that Sally is very happy, she sings and plays guitar … and is writing me a graduation song! She also said that Sally will be in the front row cheering for me … and that she is very loud. All this was getting to me, and the picture she painted of Sally was remarkable. The woman saw Sally wearing a green cap and gown and no shoes … pink glitter painted toenails, long, unruly hair; purple and pink to match her toes. She said you couldn't see this without feeling so happy you have to smile. She said that Sally remembers a time when she took my red nail polish and spilt it on the carpet, and I took the rap for her … and that she has only good memories of her family – that she loved us all, and that she always felt loved, and there was nothing any of us could have done to prevent her death. Then the woman said, 'I'm a shit singer, but she wants me to sing a song for you.'

That was it for me. She sang, 'Three Little Birds,' from Bob Marley's Legend CD – our family spent many a trip down south or hanging out in one of our bedrooms playing it and singing along at the top of our lungs. I started crying, but not with sadness. She's ok. She really is. She's free. And apparently still a cheeky bitch … she said we should hurry up and move the shit we're holding around ourselves, cos she's tired of shouting through the fog. She loves us and misses us all. She wants us to let ourselves off the hook."

Literally, as I finalised this book another email from Annie arrived. It was short and to the point. "Hi Bill, just wanted to let you know I completed my Master's last week, I'm a Clinical Psychologist!"

I emailed back, "Congratulations, the world is a better place."

Acknowledgements

This book goes back a long way; to my early days in Glasgow, as a baby psychologist, then as a neophyte academic, before somehow becoming an Associate Professor and head of a Clinical Psychology course in Australia.

Then, the realisation that I needed to be a psychotherapist rather than just teach about it.

So a stint in the UK as Clinical Director of an Alcohol and Drug agency before surprisingly ending up as a Director, co-owner and Head of Psychotherapy in an Australian boutique private psychiatric hospital.

This book was shaped by all of the above experiences.

Lots of people have influenced my thinking and have helped shape my perspective. The greatest influence has been the patients it has been my privilege to work with. They of course remain anonymous, but thank you all.

Then there is the multitude of many excellent colleagues with whom it has been my good fortune to work with and learn from. So in historical career order, may I acknowledge the following (and I know the list is really much longer.)

I note that I don't hold any of the following responsible for the ideas in this book.

In Glasgow 1972-1986:

Dr. Gordon Claridge, Dr. Gerry Greene, Dr. Peter Kershaw, Dr. Brian Riddle, Dr. Mike Dow, Prof. David Cooke, Mr. Adrian Davies, the late Prof. John Booth Davies (who wanted the words "none the wiser" on his grave stone, but thanks to you John we all are), Dr. Phil Davies, Prof. Harry Sheldon and Prof. Steve Allsop.

In Perth, Western Australia 1986-1998:

Dr. John O'Connor, Prof. Dennis Glencross, Dr. Geoff Richards and very importantly, Dr. Ali Marsh and Ms. Tania Towers who both in the early 1990s cajoled me to include developmental trauma in my work.

Then being a clinician 1998-current: Dr. John Edwards for on-going encouragement, keeping me alive and with Dr. Steven Proud (psychiatrist and protagonist) getting me involved in what turned out to be the best part of my career. Thanks guys.

And the best ever psychotherapist mate, Dr. Marc Joffe, for twenty plus years of running, psychological support, psychoanalytical wisdom and for always being kind while giving me much needed corrective guidance.

Then there is the book itself. First acknowledgement is to my wife, Dr. Rachel Bennett, who was staunchly encouraging the idea of the book, and on my mooting the idea that I needed to go off to some isolation in order to write, was totally supportive and said, "Go for as long as you need!"

Thanks also to Sally and Clive who allowed me the use of their holiday house in a seaside hamlet some 80 kilometers north of Perth. It was a superb place to write. Then there was Mr. Steve Harvey who, while walking The South Coast Pathway in the UK, listened and very helpfully advised on the nature of the book, read the early, middle and later drafts and was totally encouraging throughout. Thanks very much Steve.

And now, a bit more specifically related to the book itself, thanks to my namesake colleague Caroline Saunders for finding me a publisher, Mrs. Vanessa Neri for reading the whole thing and telling me some bits were "gold," and Ms. Jo Tedeschi for her delightful enthusiasm for the book and her technical help. Plus Dr. Clement Extier, my daughter Amelia and my wife, for coming up with a prototype book cover that was then enhanced and made real by the team at KMD publishing.

And very heartfelt thanks to Karen McDermott of KMD publishing who, within twenty-four hours of receiving a draft of the book said, "I love it!"

Music to any author's ears.

But the final accolade and thanks go to Tracey Regan for being the editor. You only realise how important an editor is when you send her a finally perfected chapter and it comes back with fifty-nine corrections and it reads better. Thanks Tracey.

Glossary

Aberrant
Departing from an accepted standard.

Aetiology
The study of the causes of a disease.

Akathisia
Movement disorder, characterised by a feeling of inner restlessness or inability to sit still.

Alleles
Two or more alternative forms of a gene that arise by mutation.

Amalgam
A mixture or blend.

Ameliorate
Make (something bad or unsatisfactory) better.

Artifice
Clever or cunning devices or expedients, especially as used to trick or deceive others.

Avolition
A lack of interest or engagement in goal-directed behaviour.

Catatonia
A group of symptoms usually involving a lack of movement and communication. Can include agitation, confusion, restlessness.

Chronocity
The state of being chronic, having a long duration.

Corallary
A proposition that follows from one already proved.

Dissociation
The action of disconnecting or separating – or the state of being disconnected.

Dyskinesias
Involuntary, erratic, writhing movements of the face, arms, legs or trunk. Often fluid, they can all be rapid jerking, or slow extended muscle spasms.

Dystonia
A movement disorder where a person's muscles contract uncontrollably.

Enervating
Causing one to feel drained of energy or vitality.

Epidemiology
The branch of medicine which deals with the incidence, distribution and possible control of diseases.

Epithet
An adjective or phrase expressing an attributor or characteristic of a person or thing.

Epiphenomena
A secondary effect or by-product.

Gerundive
Functioning as an adjective meaning 'that should or must be done'.

Hegemony
Leadership or dominance, especially by one state or social group over others.

Inculcate
Instill an idea or habit by persistent instruction.

Inimical
Tending to obstruct or harm.

Inter-rater
The extent to which two or more raters (or observers, coders, examiners) agree.

Inveigle
Persuade someone to do something by means of deception or flattery.

Malfeasant
A person who transgresses moral or civil law.

Mnemonic
A system such as a pattern of letters, ideas, or associations which assists in remembering something.

Morass
An area of muddy or boggy ground.

Neophyte
A person who is new to a subject or activity.

Nomenclature
The devising or choosing of names for things.

Non Sequitur
A conclusion or statement that does not logically follow from the previous statement.

Perjorative
Expressing contempt or disapproval.

Perspicacious
Having a ready insight into and understanding of things.

Posited
Put forward as fact, or the basis of an argument.

Psychopharmacological
The scientific study of the effects drugs have on mood, sensation, thinking, and behavior. It is distinguished from neuropsychopharmacology, which emphasizes the correlation between drug-induced changes in the functioning of cells in the nervous system and changes in consciousness and behavior.

Psychotherapy
The treatment of mental disorder by psychological rather than medical means.

Putative
Commonly put forth or accepted as true.

Tardive Dyskinesia
Stiff jerky movements of the face and body.

Trenchant
Vigorous or incisive in expression or style.

Zeitgeist
The defining spirit or mood of a particular period of history as shown by the ideas and beliefs of the time.

References

Chapter 1

- https://www.jeffreyliebermanmd.com/bio
- Bentall, R., 2009. Doctoring the mind. New York: New York University Press.
- Burstow, B., 2015. Psychiatry and the business of madness. Basingstoke: Palgrave Macmillan.
- Freedman, R., Lewis, D., Michels, R., Pine, D., Schultz, S., Tamminga, C., Gabbard, G., Gau, S., Javitt, D., Oquendo, M., Shrout, P., Vieta, E. and Yager, J., 2013. The Initial Field Trials of DSM-5: New Blooms and Old Thorns. American Journal of Psychiatry, 170(1), pp.1-5.
- Hyler, S., 1982. Reliability in the DSM-III Field Trials. Archives of General Psychiatry, 39(11), p.1275.
- Kirk, S. and Kutchins, H., 1992. The selling of DSM. New Brunswick New Jersey: Transaction Publishers.
- Lambourne, J. and Gill, D., 1978. A Controlled Comparison of Simulated and Real ECT. British Journal of Psychiatry, 133(6), pp.514-519.
- Lieberman, J., 2015. Shrinks. Croydon: Weidenfeld & Nicolson.
- Rogers, A., 2021. Star Neuroscientist Tom Insel Leaves the Google-Spawned Verily for ... a Startup?. [online] Wired. Available at: <https://www.wired.com/2017/05/star-neuroscientist-tom-insel-leaves-google-spawned-verily-startup/> [Accessed 9 April 2021].
- Rose, N., 2019. Our psychiatric future. Cambridge: Polity press.
- Rosenhan, D., 1973. On Being Sane in Insane Places. Science, 179(4070), pp.250-258.
- Scull, A., 2019. Psychiatry and its Discontents Oakland: University of California Press
- Seierstad, A., 2015. One of Us: The Story of a Massacre in Norway. London: Virago.
- Sharpe, L., Gurland, B., Fleiss, J., Kendell, R., Cooper, J. and Copeland,

- J., 1974. Comparisons of American, Canadian and British Psychiatrists in Their Diagnostic Concepts. Canadian Psychiatric Association Journal, 19(3), pp.235-245.
- Shedler, J., 2010. The efficacy of psychodynamic psychotherapy. American Psychologist, 65(2), pp.98-109.
- Spiegel, A., 2004. The dictionary of disorder. Annals of medicine, Jan 3 2005
- Yalom, I., 1991. Love's executioner and other tales of psychotherapy. London: Penguin.

Chapter 2

- Bowlby John (1988) A Secure Base Routledge London
- Allan Schore (2015) *Affect Regulation and the Origin of the Self, Psychology press and Routledge Classic editions London*
- https://www.smithsonianmag.com/science-nature/herbert-spencer-survival-of-the-fittest-180974756/
- https://www.ncbi.nlm.nih.gov/pmc/articles/PMC6220625/
- https://developingchild.harvard.edu/
- http://danielhughes.org/
- http://lizmullinar.com.au
- V J Felitti 1, R F Anda, D Nordenberg, D F Williamson, A M Spitz, V Edwards, M P Koss, J S Marks Relationship of childhood abuse and household dysfunction to many of the leading causes of death in adults. The Adverse Childhood Experiences (ACE) Study 1998 May;14(4):245-58. American Journal of preventive medicine
- Wounds that time won't heal: The neurobiology of child abuse
- MH Teicher - Cerebrum, 2000
- Ryan North Empowered to Connect Podcast www.onebighappyhome.com
- Mother's affection at 8 months predicts emotional distress in adulthood J Maselko, L Kubzansky,
- L Lipsitt, S L Buka JECH Online First, published on July 26, 2010 as 10.1136/jech.2009.097873
- Hughes D.(2009) Attachment Focussed Parenting Norton New York
- Bloom S (1997) Creating Santuary:Toward the evolution of Sane Societies New York Routledge
- Bloom A & Farragher B Destroying Santuary Oxford University Press New York
- Developmental Trauma Disorder A new, rational diagnosis for children with complex trauma histories. Bessel A. van der Kolk, MD
- Ref Anthony Storr | Higher education | The Guardian

- *www.theguardian.com* › news › mar › guardianobituaries...20 Ma
- https://www.theguardian.com/news/2001/mar/20/guardianobituaries.highereducation
- Storr A, The art of Psychotherapy (2102) (2nd Edition) Taylor & Francis London
- https://www.goodreads.com/author/quotes/36033.Anthony_Storr
- https://en.wikipedia.org/wiki/Anthony_Storr

Chapter 3

- Meichhenbaum, D. Plenary Session on Trauma The Evolution of Psychotherapy Conference Dec 2012 Annaheim California.
- Herman, J (1992) Trauma and Recovery Basic Books New York
- Linehan M Cognitive Behavioral Treatment of Borderline Personality Disorder Guilford Press New York
- Bebbington, P., 2018. Sexual abuse and psychosis: The security of research findings. Schizophrenia Research, 201, pp.37-38.
- Burroughs, A., 2012. This Is How. Sydney: Pan MacMillian.
- Levine, P., 1997. Waking the tiger. Berkeley, Calif: North Atlantic Books.
- Ogden, P., Fisher, J. and Treffers, J., 2019. Sensorimotor psychotherapy. Eeserveen: Uitgeverij Mens!.
- Shapiro, F., Kaslow, F. and Maxfield, L., 2007. Handbook of EMDR and family therapy processes. Hoboken, N.J.: John Wiley & Sons.
- Strout, E., 2016. My Name is Lucy Barton. New York: Random House.
- Varese, F., Smeets, F., Drukker, M., Lieverse, R., Lataster, T., Viechtbauer, W., Read, J., van Os, J. and Bentall, R., 2012. Childhood Adversities Increase the Risk of Psychosis: A Meta-analysis of Patient-Control, Prospective- and Cross-sectional Cohort Studies. Schizophrenia Bulletin, 38(4), pp.661-671.
- Wunderink, A., Nienhuis, F., Sytema, S. and Wiersma, D., 2006. TC6B GUIDED DISCONTINUATION VERSUS MAINTENANCE TREATMENT IN REMITTED FIRST EPISODE PSYCHOSIS: RELAPSE RATES AND FUNCTIONAL OUTCOME. Schizophrenia Research, 86, p.S51.
- Yalom, I., 1991. Love's executioner and other tales of psychotherapy. London: Penguin.
- Yalom, I., 2001. The gift of therapy. London: Piatkus Books.
- Yehuda, R., Engel, S., Brand, S., Seckl, J., Marcus, S. and Berkowitz, G., 2005. Transgenerational Effects of Posttraumatic Stress Disorder in Babies of Mothers Exposed to the World Trade Center Attacks during Pregnancy. The Journal of Clinical Endocrinology & Metabolism, 90(7), pp.4115-4118.

Chapter 4

- https://www.scottdmiller.com
- evolution of psychology conference https://www.evolutionofpsychotherapy.com/?utm_term=evolution%20of%20psychotherapy-&utm_campaign=EVO+2020&utm_medium=ppc&utm_source=adwords&hsa_cam=12177559906&hsa_tgt=kwd377504926751&hsa_mt=e&hsa_ver=3&hsa_acc=3238274495&hsa_kw=evolution%20of%20psychotherapy&hsa_src=g&hsa_grp=120670004567&hsa_ad=494558243714&hsa_net=adwords&gclid=Cj0KCQiA1pyCBhCtARIsAHaY_5dGwu-9HiKiVdVycKY9jzEEy43TvWXCSpI3l4zar-NWXp-8RHYEvaTYaAiGzEALw_wcB
- (Elkin, I et al, National Institue of Mental Health Treatment of Depression Collaborative Research Program- general effectiveness of treatment Archives of General Psychiatry 46, 971-982 1989)
- Ref for NIMH study in 1989 – pg 5 – as appears to be 1985 https://jamanetwork.com/journals/jamapsychiatry/article-abstract/493541
- APA, 2012. Recognition of psychotherapy effectiveness. APA Resolution, August 2012.
- Elkin, I., 1985. NIMH Treatment of Depression Collaborative Research Program. Archives of General Psychiatry, 42(3), p.305.
- Eysenck, H., 2002. Decline and Fall of the Freudian Empire. London: Routledge.
- GROUP, P., 1998. Matching patients with alcohol disorders to treatments: Clinical implications from Project MATCH. Journal of Mental Health, 7(6), pp.589-602.
- Miller, S., 2013. Supershrinks. Key Note Address The Evolution of Psychotherapy Conference Annaheim California

Chapter 5

- https://integratedwellness.com.au/articles/three-brains/
- https://www.psychotherapynetworker.org/blog/details/48/the-triune-brain-three-brains-attempting-to-work-as
- https://www.ncbi.nlm.nih.gov/pmc/articles/PMC4006178/
- Kolk B 2015. The Body keeps the Score . London Penguin Books :
- Yehuda, R., Engel, S., Brand, S., Seckl, J., Marcus, S. and Berkowitz, G., 2005. Transgenerational Effects of Posttraumatic Stress Disorder in Babies of Mothers Exposed to the World Trade Center Attacks during Pregnancy. The Journal of Clinical Endocrinology & Metabolism, 90(7), pp.4115-4118.

Chapter 6

- https://quotefancy.com/dorothy-rowe-quotes
- https://www.blackdoginstitute.org.au/resources-support/depression/causes/
- Baumeister, R. and Tierney, J., 2011. Willpower. New York: Penguin.
- Bentall, R., 2009. Doctoring the mind. New York: New York University Press.
- Breggin, P., 2009. The Antidepressant Fact Book. Cambridge, MA: Da Capo Press.
- Davies, J., 2017. The sedated society. palgrave macmillian.
- Edwards, G. and Grant, M., 1980. Alcoholism treatment in transition. London: Croom Helm.
- Gotzsche, P., 2017. Psychopharmacology is not evidence based medicine. In: J. Davies, ed., The Sedated Society. London: palgrave macmillian.
- Kirsch, I., 2008. Challenging Received Wisdom: Antidepressants and the Placebo Effect. McGill Journal of Medicine, 11(2), pp.219-22.
- Burstow, B., 2015. Psychiatry and the business of madness. Basingstoke: Palgrave Macmillan.
- Healy, D., 2016. Psychiatric drugs explained. 6th ed. London: Elsevier.

Chapter 8

- BENTALL ., R., 2003. Madness explained psychosis and human nature. London: Penguin.
- Breggin, P., 2017. Neuroleptic (antipsychotic) Drugs : An epidemic of tardive dyskinesia and related brain injuries afflicting tens of millions. In: J. Davies, ed., The Sedated Society. London: palgrave macmillian.
- Davies, J., 2017. The sedated society. London palgrave macmillian.
- Dutton, K., 2012. The wisdom of psychopaths. London: Heinemann.
- Gotzsche, P., 2017. Psychopharmacology is not evidence based medicine. In: J. Davies, ed., The Sedated Society. London: palgrave macmillian.
- Healy, D., 2016. Psychiatric drugs explained. 6th ed. London: Elsevier.
- Lieberman, J., 2015. Shrinks. Croydon: Weidenfeld & Nicolson.
- Messman-Moore, T. and Long, P., 2003. The role of childhood sexual abuse sequelae in the sexual revictimization of women. Clinical Psychology Review, 23(4), pp.537-571.
- Wunderink, A., Nienhuis, F., Sytema, S. and Wiersma, D., 2006. TC6B GUIDED DISCONTINUATION VERSUS MAINTENANCE TREATMENT IN REMITTED FIRST EPISODE PSYCHOSIS: RELAPSE

RATES AND FUNCTIONAL OUTCOME. Schizophrenia Research, 86, p.S51.

Chapter 9
- Burroughs, A., 2012. This Is How. Sydney: Pan MacMillian.

Chapter 10
- Dutton, K., 2012. The wisdom of psychopaths. London: Heinemann.
- Storr, A., 2015. Art of psychotherapy. London: Routledge.

Chapter 11
- Burroughs, A., 2012. This Is How. Sydney: Pan MacMillian.
- Storr, A., 2015. Art of psychotherapy. London: Routledge.
- Yalom, I., 2001. The gift of therapy. London: Piatkus Books.

Chapter 13
- Davies, J., 1997. The myth of addiction. Amsterdam, Netherlands: Harwood Academic Publishers.
- King, S., 2013. Night shift. New York: Anchor Books.
- Thomas, C. and Fazio, F., 2008. My life with Dylan Thomas. London: Virago.

Chapter 15
- Trends in injury deaths, Australia 1999–00 to 2016–17 Australian Institute of Helath and Welfare
- ISBN: 978 1 76054 650 2
- Cat. no: INJCAT 207

Chapter 16
- Rowe, D., 2003. Depression. Philadelphia, Pa.: Brunner-Routledge.

Chapter 18
- Storr, A., 1997. Solitude. London: HarperCollins.

Chapter 19

- https://www.psychologytoday.com/us/blog/side-effects/201902/our-psychiatric-future
- Burstow, B., 2015. Psychiatry and the business of madness. Basingstoke: Palgrave Macmillan. P264
- Montagu, L., 2017. Desperate for a fix: My Story of Pharmaceutical Misadventure. In: J. Davies, ed., The sedated society. palgrave macmillian. P120
- Kinderman, P., 2017. A Manifesto for Psychological Health and Wellbeing. In: J. Davies, ed., The Sedated Society. London: palgrave macmillian. P272
- Taylor, B., 2015. The Last Asylum. London: Penguin Books. P259
- Rose, N., 2019. Our psychiatric future. Cambridge: Polity press. P132 Greenberg G The Book of Woe: The DSM and the Unmaking of Psychiatry Blue Rider Press, 2013

www.ingramcontent.com/pod-product-compliance
Lightning Source LLC
Chambersburg PA
CBHW021404290426
44108CB00010B/380